RECONSTRUCTING MEANING AFTER TRAUMA

RECONSTRUCTING MEANING AFTER TRAUMA
Theory, Research, and Practice

Edited by

ELIZABETH M. ALTMAIER

Amsterdam • Boston • Heidelberg • London
New York • Oxford • Paris • San Diego
San Francisco • Singapore • Sydney • Tokyo

Academic Press is an imprint of Elsevier

Academic Press is an imprint of Elsevier
125 London Wall, London EC2Y 5AS, United Kingdom
525 B Street, Suite 1800, San Diego, CA 92101-4495, United States
50 Hampshire Street, 5th Floor, Cambridge, MA 02139, United States
The Boulevard, Langford Lane, Kidlington, Oxford OX5 1GB, United Kingdom

Library of Congress Cataloging-in-Publication Data
A catalog record for this book is available from the Library of Congress

British Library Cataloguing-in-Publication Data
A catalogue record for this book is available from the British Library

ISBN: 978-0-12-803015-8

For information on all Academic Press publications
visit our website at http://www.elsevier.com/

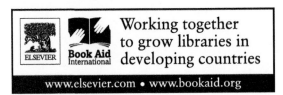

Working together
to grow libraries in
developing countries

www.elsevier.com • www.bookaid.org

Publisher: Nicky Levy
Acquisition Editor: Emily Ekle
Editorial Project Manager: Timothy Bennett
Production Project Manager: Lisa Jones
Designer: Matthew Limbert

CONTENTS

Part 2 Mechanisms of Meaning Loss and Restoration

LIST OF CONTRIBUTORS

K. Adams
Caboolture Regional Domestic Violence Service, Caboolture, QLD, Australia

G.E.K. Allen
Brigham Young University, Provo, UT, United States

M. Baker
University of Minnesota, Minneapolis, MN, United States

R.E. Bernstein
University of Oregon, Eugene, OR, United States

P.J. Birrell
Independent Practitioner, Eugene, OR, United States

C.J. Bryan
The University of Utah, Salt Lake City, UT, United States

C.J. Button
United States Air Force, Little Rock Air Force Base, AR, United States

C.A. Courtois
Independent Practice, (retired), Washington, DC, United States

P. Frazier
University of Minnesota, Minneapolis, MN, United States

J.J. Freyd
University of Oregon, Eugene, OR, United States

A.C. Hoffman
University of Iowa, Iowa City, IA, United States; University of Illinois at Urbana-Champaign, Champaign, IL, United States

J. Jinkerson
Fielding Graduate University, Santa Barbara, CA, United States; Air Force Institute of Technology, OH, United States

B.K. Jones
Northwestern University, Evanston, IL, United States

M.A. Keitel
Fordham University, New York, NY, United States

M.C. Kennedy
Philadelphia University, Philadelphia, PA, United States

T. Lea
Brigham Young University, Provo, UT, United States

K. Lipari
Fordham University, New York, NY, United States

D.P. McAdams
Northwestern University, Evanston, IL, United States

M.A. Meyer DeMott
University College of South East Norway, Oslo, Norway; Norwegian Institute for Expressive Arts and Communications, Oslo, Norway; European Graduate School, Saas Fee, Switzerland

V. Nguyen-Feng
University of Minnesota, Minneapolis, MN, United States

C.L. Park
University of Connecticut, Storrs, CT, United States

P.S. Richards
Brigham Young University, Provo, UT, United States

M. Schenkenfelder
Iowa State University, Ames, IA, United States

J.M. Schultz
Augustana College, Rock Island, IL, United States

J. Shakespeare-Finch
Queensland University of Technology, Brisbane, QLD, Australia

B.A. Tallman
Coe College, Cedar Rapids, IA, United States; UnityPoint Health-St. Luke's Hospital, Cedar Rapids, IA, United States

N. Wade
Iowa State University, Ames, IA, United States

H. Wertz
Fordham University, New York, NY, United States

INTRODUCTION
MEANING AND CONNECTION AFTER TRAUMA

E.M. Altmaier

Research and clinical work is currently being transformed by the recognition that many people have past trauma histories that influence their present lives. Within research, scholars are considering topics that expand previous views of trauma. Examples of that expansion are new concepts of trauma, such as betrayal trauma (Freyd, 1996); increased assessment of adverse childhood events in the study of adolescent or adult psychosocial issues; and new attention to various types of trauma, such as military sexual trauma. There are well-developed specific treatments for trauma, but some clients may be seeking help for a problem that is not directly related to a trauma in their past. However, their concerns must be addressed within a trauma-informed environment. Clinically, trauma-informed treatment is not a particular approach, but rather an adherence to principles that maintain safety, trustworthiness, peer support, collaboration, empowerment, and cultural integrity within any treatment.

Recovery, whether from trauma or within a context partially formed by prior trauma, is the ultimate goal of treatment. Recovery, however, is difficult to define. Is recovery merely the absence of symptoms that led to the diagnosis or to the treatment? In a parallel manner, would we define health merely as the absence of illness? Our own personal experience and expert scholarship combine in our knowing that health is much more than the absence of a negative; it is the presence of many positives. Recovery, therefore, is more than the absence of the "negatives" of trauma; it is the presence of many positives.

Leamy, Bird, Le Boutillier, Williams, and Slade (2011) completed a thematic analysis of studies on recovery and discovered specific characteristics shared by various approaches to recovery. First, recovery is individual and unique: no one person's recovery serves as a ready-made template for the recovery of another. Second, recovery can occur in the absence of a "cure." Third, and relevant for this book, recovery is a struggle. Recovery takes effort, commitment, strength, courage, and passion. Fourth, recovery is not a linear process. Rather, it is irregular, with steps forward, and steps backward, and time away from the process. Last, recovery involves many series of trials and errors to accomplish. That which was successful in one phase of recovery may not be successful in another.

Brown (2012) writes movingly of the process of "daring greatly." Her book title is taken from a speech given by Theodore Roosevelt in Paris in 1910. To recover, people must take on a stance of vulnerability. This stance was articulated by Roosevelt as follows:

> It is not the critic who counts; not the man who points out how the strong man stumbles, or where the doer of deeds could have done them better. The credit belongs to the man who is actually in the arena, whose face is marred by dust and sweat and blood; who strives valiantly; who errs, who comes short again and again, because there is no effort without error or shortcoming; but who does actually strive to do the deeds; who knows great enthusiasms, the great devotions; who spends himself in a worthy cause; who at the best knows in the end the triumph of high achievement, and who at the worst, if he fails, at least fails while daring greatly.

Recovery after trauma requires this degree of effort, vulnerability, and spending of oneself because to succeed, recovery must have the following resources.

Recovery requires **connectedness**. Isolation after trauma removes us from necessary emotional and instrumental support we receive from other people. Being part of a community of recovering individuals has been valued for many forms of recovery. However, for persons after trauma, interpersonal connectedness is often impaired.

Recovery requires **storytelling**. Recreating meaning in the iterative narrative process is storytelling, and stories are told by one person to another. Connectedness to another creates the climate of trust in which storytelling can occur. But traumatized individuals are reluctant to re-visit their traumas, and avoidance or denial is a frequent coping response.

Recovery requires **hope** and optimism about the future. To stick with the tasks of recovery, there must be a likelihood of change, a dream of a new possible self, and hopefulness in a present that supports confidence in change. Making a new meaning is the lens of hope put to the past that creates a fresh and different vision of the future. However, trauma shatters the hope of many. Restoring this hope in the face of circumstances that cannot be changed is a primary need for traumatized persons.

Recovery means building a new **identity**. That new identity will be clear of shame, of stigma, of betrayal. Building a new identity will be a collage of past selves, current selves, and possible future selves. Its assembly is an artistic, creative endeavor. For persons after trauma, their prior selves, with their beliefs and core assumptions, are gone. Therefore, to remake an identity is a challenging task that requires time and purpose.

Recovery will be firmly rooted in **meaning**. Meaning will permeate all aspects of life, from social, personal, spiritual, to vocational. New meaning structures will be spoken into being, and will scaffold the building of the new identity and the new future. Trauma, by its nature, shatters prior meaning. Rebuilding meaning after trauma is the core issue of recovery, and the focus of this book.

Recovery requires personal **empowerment**. Empowerment is the stamina of personal resolve. It includes responsibility for recovery, for one's responses to circumstances and situations whether controllable or not controllable, and a clear vision of one's own strengths. Trauma, however, reduces empowerment to impotence. Assisting traumatized individuals to reclaim and regain their power and competence is a necessary goal of treatment.

The chapters in this book were chosen with one aim: to give the practicing clinician knowledge and skills to incorporate meaning making into the treatment of clients after trauma. Although recent publications (see Markman, Prouix, & Lindberg, 2013) have provided groundbreaking work on scholarship in the growing field of meaning, the translation of that work to the day-to-day lives of clinicians in their practices is less available. In the present text, that was the challenge to each of the authors. How can the growing theory and research on meaning making be translated into applications for the practicing clinician? What is new knowledge about the nature of trauma and meaning? What are the mechanisms by which meaning can be restored? What is important to know about specific traumatized populations: victims of sexual assault, persons with ongoing exposure to trauma such as emergency medical responders, persons with acquired disability, refugees and exiles, and combat survivors?

Reconstructing Meaning after Trauma: Theory, Research and Practice has intentionally used a specific chapter structure where a case is presented, and then analyzed within the theory, research, and clinical recommendations of that chapter. Chapter authors were selected for their expertise in the chapter topic. Chapters were written to be understandable to a variety of professional providers who work with traumatized clients, across a global scale. Three specific sections of the book are defined.

The first section provides foundational material on the two major topics of the book: meaning and trauma. Dan McAdams and Brady Jones consider the paradox that trauma shatters meaning and creates distress for many persons, but not all. They describe resilience, and discuss characteristics of resilient persons. They also cover processes by which persons who suffer from trauma rebuild their personal meanings through such means as sense making and benefit finding. Crystal Park and Christine Kennedy then provide a complete model of how people have both global beliefs and situational beliefs, and concurrent violations of these beliefs after trauma. These violations promote cognitive and emotional processing to restore the concordance of situational and global meanings. Last, Pamela Birrell, Rosemary Bernstein, and Jennifer Freyd expand the individualistic view of trauma to a connectedness view, and flesh out the violations of trauma that occurs within a relational connection. In this case, the trauma damages or betrays both the individual and the relational context, which may be an institution or a social system. Traumas higher in betrayal have more several consequences, and may be a cause of "betrayal blindness," a concept that explains why traumatized individuals are in great danger of being retraumatized.

The second section considers specific influences on both the experience of trauma and the restoration of meaning. This section seeks to consider personal characteristics that might affect the ways in which the foundation models described in the first section operate. Two such characteristics are gender and culture. Merle Keitel, Kristen Lipari, and Hannah Wertz consider gender in the specific trauma of cancer diagnosis and treatment. The role of culture, and its contributions, are explored by Kawika Allen, Scott Richards, and Troy Lea. They also focus on characteristics of specific cultures in responding to trauma. In addition, although there are likely many mechanisms of meaning restoration, interpersonal trauma created by the wounding of one person by another has often been linked with forgiveness as a means of responding to the trauma. Nathaniel Wade, Jessica Schultz, and Mary Schenkenfelder describe forgiveness in its unprompted forms as well as treatments that promote forgiveness within a meaning-making focus.

Trauma occurs for many specific populations. For this book, the final section on special populations focuses on five populations and varying treatment modalities. Patricia Frazier, Therese Bermingham, Viann Nguyen-Feng, and Majel Baker consider components of meaning making following sexual assault, including meanings that may impede growth such as self-blame. They also define treatments that allow sexual assault survivors to reduce fear and change event meaning. An often unexplored population is introduced by Jane Shakespeare-Finch and Kay Adams, that of emergency medical dispatchers who vicariously participate in the trauma of others. To assist victims, these persons must bring to mind the trauma scene, including sounds, sights, and environment. The global belief that the world is a safe place is continually violated within their work life, and Shakespeare-Finch and Adams discuss how the sense of coherence helps with meaning making.

As our population ages, older (and younger) people experience an acquired disability. This new physical or mental impairment creates major disruptions in function, particularly activities of daily living. Benjamin Tallman and Anna Hoffman revisit a theme from the first chapter, that of the paradox of some persons showing great resilience whereas, in similar circumstances, others experience deep distress and depression. Tallman and Hoffman consider how these disabling circumstances can work to foster posttraumatic growth, improvements in self-perception, relationships, spirituality and faith, and plans for the future.

On a global scale, refugees and exiles from home are increasing dramatically. These persons have lives that are trauma filled. Melinda Ashley Meyer DeMott introduces the use of expressive arts, and presents a range of non-verbally mediated ways of reconstructing meaning, particularly within connection to others. In a related vein, on a global scale, combat in many forms is increasing. Combat-related trauma is especially difficult within the military culture, which espouses a warrior ethos. Christopher Button, Jeremy Jinkerson, and Craig Bryan explore both lost meanings and moral injuries, and how global beliefs and meaning can be restored.

In the final section, Christine Courtois serves a complex role in her chapter that unites and integrates the chapters in the book. Courtois moves back from the specifics of individual influences and populations to revisit notions of trauma, treatment, and meaning restoration. In a role similar to that of a symposium discussant, Courtois brings her own expertise to the book and allows us to reconsider the book's themes and content from her perspectives.

This book is predicated on the notion that meaning is a movement from a word or group of words to an interpretation. Across time, these interpretations gain power and form structure in our perceptual lives. That definition parallels that of Personal Construct Theory, a before-his-time contribution by George Kelly during the 1950s. Kelly (1955) believed that a person's psychological processes are "channeled" by how he or she anticipates events. We use "constructs" to complete that anticipation process.

This early statement of constructivism is repeated in current studies of meaning. When some aspect of our own experience forces us to work to understand it, either for the first time or in a new way, our cognitive processes search for similarity. Thus metaphor often undergirds meaning. Common metaphors are "life is a journey," "life is a path." Consider the many meanings that are packed within a metaphor such as life is a journey. A journey requires planning, acquiring resources, determining whether sufficient resources exist, making a beginning, experiencing delays and setbacks, getting lost and getting back on track, getting help from travel companions, and arriving at a destination.

Meanings do more than simply "pile up" like a cord of wood. Rather, they serve in a developmental transformative way, shaking apart and reforming our lives through our perceptions, our constructions, and our responses to both positive and negative events. Trauma, by definition, violently shatters our meanings and thus requires considerable effort to rebuild. The authors of this book contribute in an exceptional way to our efforts as clinicians to understand and to participate and to facilitate our clients' meaning making in the wake of trauma.

REFERENCES

Brown, B. (2012). *Daring greatly: How the courage to be vulnerable transforms the way we live, love, parent, and lead*. New York: Penguin Group.

Freyd, J. (1996). *Betrayal trauma: The logic of forgetting childhood abuse*. Cambridge, MA: Harvard University Press.

Kelly, G. A. (1955). *The psychology of personal constructs*. New York: Norton. 2 volumes.

Leamy, M., Bird, V., Le Boutillier, C., Williams, J., & Slade, M. (2011). Conceptual framework for personal recovery in mental health: a systematic review and narrative synthesis. *The British Journal of Psychiatry, 199*, 445–452.

Markman, K. D., Proulx, T., & Lindberg, M. J. (Eds.). (2013). *The psychology of meaning*. Washington, DC: American Psychological Association.

PART 1

Foundations of Meaning and Trauma

CHAPTER 1

Making Meaning in the Wake of Trauma: Resilience and Redemption

D.P. McAdams, B.K. Jones
Northwestern University, Evanston, IL, United States

Shortly after his release from a Nazi concentration camp, Viktor Frankl spent nine fevered days composing an account of the harrowing experiences he endured in Dachau and Auschwitz. What he first conceived to be an anonymous report eventually became the basis for one of the most celebrated books of the 20th century. In *Man's Search for Meaning*, Frankl (1959/1992) forged an immutable link between trauma and meaning. The quest for meaning is a fundamental human propensity, Frankl argued. And traumatic events in life—even the horrific suffering that Frankl and countless others experienced in the Holocaust—invoke the search for meaning in two ways. First, trauma violently shakes people out of their conventions and their comfort zones, refocusing their consciousness on existential questions of life. You do not have to suffer greatly to reflect upon the meaning of your life, but suffering can jump-start or accelerate the process. Second, trauma can violate or undermine sacrosanct assumptions about human life, challenging the victim or survivor to formulate new meanings. Under extreme conditions, the failure to sustain old meanings or create new ones in the wake of trauma can threaten survival. Prisoners who lost meaning simply gave up and died at Auschwitz.

Beyond the unspeakable physical privations and losses that Frankl suffered in the camps, his bedrock presuppositions about human nature and the world were obliterated. A well-educated Jew who figured to find a productive niche one day in a highly civilized society, Frankl came to witness instead unmitigated evil and a devastating meltdown of the social order. In the terms of one contemporary expert on trauma and meaning, Frankl experienced the shattering of two of three fundamental assumptions about life: (1) that the world is benevolent and (2) that justice or fairness prevails

Reconstructing Meaning After Trauma
ISBN 978-0-12-803015-8
http://dx.doi.org/10.1016/B978-0-12-803015-8.00001-2

(Janoff-Bulman, 1992). He seemed even to question the third assumption—that the self is worthy—although perhaps not to the extent of ever completely losing hope in his own agency. Like many Holocaust survivors, Frankl struggled to rebuild his assumptive world after the war.

Frankl's ideas derived from a singular historical moment involving countless perpetrators and millions of victims, whereas there is a sense in which psychologists' thinking about the reconstruction of meaning after trauma resembles, for each individual life, the Holocaust writ small. Whether the trauma is sexual assault, the death of a child, or a paralyzing combat wound, the expectation is that the survivor will, like Frankl, confront a crisis in meaning. The survivor may struggle to make sense of the traumatic event. Although the pain may never go away, the survivor may ultimately derive some modicum of benefit from the trauma, or from the struggle to cope with the trauma. Posttraumatic growth (PTG) may even occur (Tedeschi & Calhoun, 2004). In the wake of trauma, newfound personal strengths or enhanced interpersonal relationships or a renewed sense of spirituality may arise, suggesting that positive, growth-inducing meanings have been made. There remains the hope for redemption, albeit in an attenuated form, for the trauma itself—the disability, the assault, the murder, the nearly unbearable loss—can never be undone.

How do people make meaning in the wake of trauma? There are surely many viable answers to this question, but behind many of them is the supposition that meaning is made, in large part, through narrative. Coming from a humanistic/existentialist perspective, Neimeyer (2006) urges clinicians to help trauma victims "re-story" their lives (p. 68). Adopting the frame of cognitive behavioral therapy, Meichenbaum (2006) has developed a "constructive narrative model of posttraumatic reactions" (p. 356). He explicitly identifies story themes and plots that either promote or undermine PTG. Calhoun and Tedeschi (2001) write: "A primary task of the clinician working with people who have experienced significant loss is to assist in the process of rebuilding the damaged or shattered worldview, to help the client develop a new life narrative that incorporates the loss in a helpful way" (p. 166). Outside the clinical realm, a growing number of personality and developmental psychologists contend that human beings are storytellers by nature and that successful adaptation to negative events in life involves creating new personal narratives that affirm positive meaning in adversity (McAdams, 2006; McAdams & McLean, 2013). Pals and McAdams (2004) assert that PTG may best be understood as a process of constructing a narrative understanding of how the self has been positively transformed by the traumatic event and then integrating this transformed sense of self into an identity-defining life story.

Creating positive posttraumatic meanings through the construction of new life stories that affirm growth and human redemption would seem to resonate with Frankl's message. New stories may help to rebuild the narrator's assumptive world. The victim of a violent crime, for example, may have to abandon forever the belief that the world is benevolent, but renarrating the trauma with a focus on the people who came to his or her aid may result in a new faith in the power of human beings to support, care for, and heal one another. Clinicians may assist in the meaning reconstruction by listening carefully to their clients' stories and helping them reframe narratives in more life-affirming ways (Sheikh, 2008). But when it comes to trauma, things do not always play out in this manner. Most notably, for some people who have experienced potentially traumatic events, world assumptions may not be shattered, or even shaken, and life may proceed in a more-or-less adaptive manner. For these especially resilient people, there may indeed be no need to make new meanings.

WHEN NEW STORIES ARE NOT NEEDED: THE (SURPRISINGLY COMMON) CASE OF RESILIENCE

This chapter's first author has a friend—let us call her Laura—who, at age 32, experienced a stillborn birth and, in her early 50s, lost her husband to cancer. One of the most youthful and dashing midlife men one could ever know, Laura's husband seemed to be recovering well from his illness when she reached for him in bed one morning, and found him to be dead. On the death of her baby, Laura reported to her friends that she felt great sadness but that she refused to dwell on it. She and her husband found solace, they both reported, in reading Kushner's (1981) book, *When Bad Things Happen to Good People*. Laura got pregnant again soon after. Eventually she had three healthy children. Her husband's death, two decades later, was a shock to everybody in Laura's social circle. But Laura seemed almost unfazed. Her grieving was private and seemed relatively brief. Rather than change her life in any dramatic way after her husband died, Laura doubled down on the roles and commitments that had sustained her throughout her adult life. She drew even closer to her husband's family. She continued to care for her children. She continued to pursue the same professional, personal, and community involvements that she had enjoyed during her marriage. Nearly a decade hence, she has not dated other men, even though she has ample opportunity to do so.

We cannot be sure, of course, but Laura's case seems to defy expectations regarding (1) shattered world assumptions in the wake of trauma and (2) the subsequent construction of new, redemptive stories to promote PTG. Instead, she seems to exhibit cardinal features of what Bonanno (2004) describes as *resilience*. Reviewing a broad swath of research, Bonanno (2004) argues that many people who experience extremely negative events continue on with their lives in a more-or-less adaptive manner, exhibiting only minor and fleeting disruptions in their ability to function. He writes: "Resilient individuals may experience transient perturbations in normal functioning (e.g., several weeks of sporadic preoccupation or restless sleep) but generally exhibit a stable trajectory of healthy functioning across time, as well as the capacity for generative experiences and positive emotions" (Bonanno, 2004, p. 21).

Resilient people rarely consult clinicians because they rarely suffer the kind of psychopathology states—depression, high levels of anxiety, dissociation and psychic numbing, and other symptoms associated with post-traumatic stress disorder—that require treatment. As such, resilient individuals fly under the radar. Although exact figures are not known, Bonanno (2004) speculates that as many as 40–50% of trauma survivors may exhibit a resilience trajectory. Some skeptics might argue that resilient survivors are failing to come to terms with the trauma in their lives, boding ill for long-term adaptation, whereas Bonanno (2004) and others (e.g., Silver & Updegraff, 2013) argue the reverse. They contend that traumatic events often do not shatter assumptions, that many people do not, and need not, endure prolonged and intense grieving or distress in the wake of trauma, and that for many people there is no need to make new meanings when extremely bad things happen in their lives. Indeed the search for meaning in the wake of trauma may be akin to a fool's errand for some people, as shown in studies that link the search for meaning in trauma with heightened levels of distress (Silver & Updegraff, 2013). Instead, it may be better to put the trauma neatly behind you and move forward with your life, as Laura seems to have done.

How are resilient people able to accomplish this feat? Bonanno (2004) is careful to emphasize that resilience does not inoculate a survivor from pain and suffering. But resilient people seem to have at their disposal an arsenal of coping weapons that help them stave off traumatic assault. Among these are high levels of social support, personality dispositions that reinforce a sense of hardiness (showing courage, welcoming challenge, thriving on adversity), a tendency to engage in self-enhancement, an ability to trigger and savor positive emotions, and a repressive coping style. On the latter point, it is interesting to note that studies of Holocaust survivors suggest that some degree of repression is good for coping with trauma. In Kaminer and Lavie (1993), for example, well-adjusted survivors had lower recall of dreams related to their experiences in the concentration camps compared to survivors showing poor adjustment. For mental health workers, assisting traumatized survivors to dismiss or let go of the terrors of the past, whenever possible, may have more adaptive value, in some cases, than strategies emphasizing "working through" the trauma.

BUT MANY PEOPLE STILL NEED TO MAKE MEANING: THE PROBLEM OF SENSE MAKING

Whatever the precise prevalence of resilience turns out to be, it is clear that a sizeable number of survivors do not manifest the trajectory identified by Bonnano (2004). Characterizing their existential disillusionment in terms of "shattered" assumptions may be something of an overstatement for many (Park, 2010), whereas there is no doubt that victims of sexual assault, motor vehicle accidents, natural disasters, war atrocities, heart attacks, and other traumatic events often lose faith in the benevolence of humankind, the fairness of society, and/or the worthiness of the self (Janoff-Bulman, 1992). Different kinds of trauma pose different kinds of challenges in meaning making. For example, survivors of sexual assault or abuse often lose confidence in their own worthiness and may (partly or fully) blame themselves for the assaults (Frazier, 2003). Cancer victims may be somewhat less likely to blame themselves, but they may recurrently pose the painful question, "Why me?" Many people feel the need to make sense of the negative events that have happened to them. Indeed, adversity commonly prompts and motivates a process of re-storying personal experience (McAdams & McLean, 2013; Neimeyer, 2006). In their efforts to construct coherent stories for their own lives, adolescents and adults will often try to make narrative sense of negative experiences. Adversity and trauma seem to call out for a clear narrative answer.

According to Pals (2006), the first step in constructing a meaningful narrative about personal adversity is to delve deeply into the experience, exploring and reflecting upon one's feelings, thoughts, and motivations. Along with Tedeschi and Calhoun (2004) and other proponents of PTG (e.g., Joseph & Linley, 2005), Pals (2006) suggests that deep processing of negative events in one's life may ultimately promote personal growth.

Indeed, Tedeschi and Calhoun (2004) write: "The degree to which the person is engaged cognitively by the crisis appears to be a central element in the process of posttraumatic growth" (p. 12). The introspection, cognitive engagement, and self-examination cannot go on forever, however, lest the survivor sink into obsessive and protracted rumination. Accordingly, the second step is to construct a positive resolution to the crisis, creating a redemptive narrative of the self that moves from suffering to closure (Pals, 2006). The positive resolution may leave the person with new insights or strengths, and it also serves to create the needed emotional distance from the trauma. Consistent with Pals' model, researchers who study autobiographical memory have shown that psychological adaptation tends to be positively associated with the extent to which people feel that they own and control their own memories, rather than feeling owned or controlled by the memories themselves (Beike & Crone, 2012).

Authoritative reviews of the empirical and clinical literature make it clear that many people self-consciously endeavor to find meaning in trauma (Davis, 2001; Park, 2010). But what do people really mean when they report that they are searching for meaning? Davis (2001) suggests that many people are trying to find a causal reason for the negative event. He labels this activity *sense making*. There are many different kinds of reasons that people may identify when they try to make sense of trauma. For example, they may invoke divine intervention: God was teaching me a lesson; God has a plan for my life; God works in mysterious ways. They may instead identify natural causes: My poor diet caused my cancer; the man who abused me was mentally ill. Moreover, sense making may often involve counterfactual thinking, as in wondering "what might have been" had some factor or another been different in the time or situations leading up to the traumatic event (Davis, 2001; King & Hicks, 2007).

Reviews of research on this kind of sense making reveal that many people search for but never achieve satisfying answers to their questions. For example, Silver, Boon, and Stones (1983) found that making sense of the incest they experienced still preoccupied 80% of the women in the study 10 years after the termination of the abuse. Davis, Nolen-Hoeksema, and Larson (1998) found that many parents who suffered the loss of a child to sudden infant death syndrome said that it was important to make some cognitive and emotional sense of the event, but most reported never being able to find meaning. Those parents who reported never searching at all for meaning, and indeed never finding any, showed the best adaptation to the loss. Moreover, reviews show the longer a person persists in trying to make sense of trauma, the worse his or her adjustment to the trauma is likely to be (Davis, 2001; Park, 2010; Silver & Updegraff, 2013). Contra Pals (2006), and even contra Frankl (1959/1992), these findings seem to caution against any effort to make sense of trauma.

Or do they?

It should not be surprising that a lengthy period of meaning search would be associated with greater distress and poorer outcomes among trauma survivors. Silver and Updegraff (2013) observe that people who look to make sense of traumatic experiences tend to find meaning relatively quickly, within a month or so. If they are not successful by then, it is quite likely that they will never arrive at a satisfying explanation for the trauma, Silver and Updegraff (2013) assert. A long-term search, therefore, may be indicative of other problems related to the trauma, and to the survivor's life more generally, and all these are likely to bode ill. Moreover, when people report that they do manage to find meaning, even after a protracted search, their psychological health usually improves (Park, 2010). Among cancer survivors, for example, deriving satisfactory meanings from the illness has been shown to predict positive outcomes concurrently and later on (Park, Edmondson, Fenster, & Blank, 2008). The bottom line is that resilient people may not need to engage in substantive sense making in the wake of trauma. But for the rest of us, successful recovery may depend, in part, on being able to construct a sensible explanation for the meaning and significance of the trauma.

What counts for a sensible explanation will vary widely from one person to the next. Davis's (2001) conception of sense making focuses narrowly on causal explanations for events. Making sense of the trauma effectively means figuring out how, and why, it came to be. But the kinds of meanings people make out of negative events in their lives cover a much more expansive psychological topography. For Pals (2006), the first step in constructing a redemptive narrative about trauma is to examine one's feelings, thoughts, and motivations related to the negative event, not necessarily to figure out how the event came to be, but instead to understand how the event has affected you and what role it plays in your ongoing life narrative. In describing clinical interventions with bereaved parents, Klass (2001) argues that the "goal of grief is not to sever the bond with the dead child but to integrate the child into the parent's life and social networks in a different way than when the child was alive" (p. 77). In an especially intriguing insight, Klass suggests that the memory of their dead child functions as a reminder for parents of how they need to live worthy lives going forward. In this powerful form of meaning making, the child becomes an internalized and symbolized "teacher of life's important lessons" (Klass, 2001, p. 90). Finally, Park (2010) enumerates a litany of different ways that people claim to make meaning out of trauma, including the sense making that comes with causal understandings, of course, and also acceptance, changed identity, changed global beliefs, changed global goals, and perception of growth or positive life changes. Her last example, finding benefit and positive change in suffering, goes to the heart of what researchers and clinicians have repeatedly described as PTG.

WHEN BAD THINGS RESULT IN GOOD THINGS: BENEFIT FINDING IN THE WAKE OF TRAUMA

The idea that suffering may ultimately result in enhancement has ancient roots. As James (1902/1958) noted in *The Varieties of Religious Experience*, all the world's great religions begin with the problem of human suffering. Suffering originates in human flaws or frailties of some sort, or in the very nature of human existence. Thus, Christians and Jews speak of original sin, whereas Buddhists ascribe suffering to *dukkha*, which denotes universal human conflict and sorrow. Each religious tradition suggests what human beings need to do or experience in order to be delivered from suffering to a positive state. In the Christian tradition, the move is from sin to salvation, which ultimately derives, Christian doctrine maintains, from the crucifixion and resurrection of Jesus Christ. The trauma of Christ's death paves the way for the spiritual (and bodily) benefits that Christians may enjoy. In a parallel fashion, each Christian life may chart its own journey of redemption, be it through a process of growth and the deepening of faith or through a sudden transformation, as in religious conversion.

Religious traditions typically aim to instill hope and optimism in their followers, whereas the movement from suffering to enhancement also appears in the timeless genre of tragedy. Take the ancient Greek myth of Oedipus. The protagonist's fate seems relentlessly harsh in *Oedipus Rex*: because he (unknowingly) killed his father and (unknowingly) slept with his mother, Oedipus is blinded and banished from the city. When the truth of parricide and incest is finally revealed, Oedipus must resign himself to his destiny, paying the price for his (unwitting) hubris. But the myth does not end here. In subsequent stories (e.g., *Oedipus at Colonus*), Oedipus returns to his people in the role of a wise sage and peacemaker.

In developing the idea of the Oedipus Complex, Freud charted the same move in psychodynamic narrative. Like Oedipus, the young child must suffer a harsh defeat, although on an unconscious level. The child ultimately renounces unconscious longings for sexual union and succumbs to, while identifying with, the aggressive authority who stands in the way of wish fulfillment. As a result, the post-Oedipal child internalizes a superego, which marks the genesis, Freud insisted, of a moral sensibility in the psyche. You do not have to buy into Freud's theory to appreciate the narrative arc: Suffering leads to enhancement, as the young protagonist ultimately experiences growth and obtains psychological benefits in the wake of the Oedipal defeat. Freud believed that the tragedy of Oedipus, enacted on a private, unconscious stage, strips the child of a destructive psychological hubris, and thereby prepares him or her for positive interpersonal relationships in a moral community. It is no coincidence, in this regard, that literary scholars, mental health workers, and many laypeople recognize the power of tragedy to bring people together (Alon & Omer, 2004).

When it comes to the psychological literature on meaning making, many scholars distinguish between sense making and benefit finding (e.g., Davis, 2001). In benefit finding, a person identifies the emergence of a newfound strength or attribute that results from a negative experience. In the area of health psychology, studies have shown, for instance, that when people who suffer heart attacks explicitly identify a benefit that they believe has resulted from their illness (such as a greater appreciation for life or improved relationships with loved ones), they tend to enjoy a better prognosis down the road (e.g., they are less likely to suffer a second heart attack), compared with cardiac patients who do not perceive a benefit in their illness (Affleck & Tennen, 1996). As an especially salutary form of making meaning, benefit finding enjoys an exalted status in the trauma literature. Interestingly, benefit finding seems to point to cognitive and emotional processes that may be independent of those putatively associated with sense making (Davis, 2001). Research suggests that the tendency to engage in benefit finding is uncorrelated with sense making. Moreover, although sense making appears to decline over time following a trauma, benefit finding appears to increase with time (Davis, 2001).

Benefit finding is at the center of what many clinicians and researchers describe as the broader phenomenon of PTG. Tedeschi and Calhoun (2004) define PTG as:

> *the experience of positive change that occurs as a result of the struggle with highly challenging life circumstances. It is manifested in a variety of ways, including an increased appreciation for life in general, more meaningful interpersonal relationships, an increased sense of personal strength, changed priorities, and richer existential and spiritual life. (p. 1)*

Reports of PTG have been documented in bereavement, heart attacks, cancer, spinal cord injury, multiple sclerosis, infertility, natural disasters, transportation accidents, rape, military combat, chemical dependency, and refugee experiences, among other traumas and negative events (Joseph & Linley, 2005; Tedeschi & Calhoun, 2004). From the standpoint of personal narratives, PTG represents a successful effort to construct a redemptive story around personal trauma (Calhoun & Tedeschi, 2001; Neimeyer, 2006; Pals & McAdams, 2004). A growing body of research in personality and developmental psychology shows that the tendency to construct redemptive stories about life is associated with psychological well-being, psychosocial maturity, and prosocial civic engagement (McAdams, 2006; McAdams & Guo, 2015). Redemptive stories appear to promote well-being in the face of collective trauma, as well. Adler and Poulin (2009) found that Americans who derived redemptive meaning from the 9/11 attacks, and who indicated greater levels of positive psychological closure in their narrative accounts of 9/11, had higher scores on psychological well-being than those Americans whose stories of 9/11 lacked clear positive resolutions.

It should be noted, however, that successful PTG needs to go beyond the realm of personal narrative and meaning making to involve demonstrable change in a person's social behavior and emotional experience. Real growth in the wake of trauma may begin with changed meanings, but it should also be reflected in improved performance of social roles, enhanced commitments, and observable behavior in the service of positive goals. Meaning may inform behavior, but meaning and behavior are still two different things. In this light, there is some evidence in the research literature to suggest that subjective, retrospective assessments of PTG may not exactly correspond to objectively assessed change in people's social and emotional functioning (Frazier et al., 2009). In the wake of trauma, many people may believe they have experienced growth. Determining whether or not they actually have achieved growth, however, should probably go beyond merely taking their word for it.

COMMUNITY AND CULTURE: MEANING MAKING IS ALWAYS SOCIAL AND LOCAL

Empirical researchers who study meaning making in the wake of trauma usually take as their unit of analysis the individual meaning maker himself or herself. But clinicians, mental health workers, and the trauma survivors themselves know that meaning making happens within a specific human community and in the context of ongoing interpersonal relationships. (Researchers know this, too, but they find it difficult to design studies that take so many specific factors into consideration.) More broadly, the whole business of constructing life narratives to make sense and meaning out of personal experiences—be it everyday experiences or traumatic events—is a deeply and complexly social process, strongly shaped by cultural norms (Hammack, 2008; McAdams, 2006). We are coauthors of our own life stories at best, and shameless plagiarists.

Clinically informed sources tend to emphasize the social and cultural dimensions of meaning making in the wake of trauma (e.g., Etherington, 2008; Klass, 2001; Neimeyer, 2006; Sheikh, 2008; Weiss & Berger, 2010). It is well recognized that social support tends to promote successful recovery from trauma (Ozer, Best, Lipsey, & Weiss, 2003). Beyond encouraging their clients to seek help from friends and family members, however, clinicians need to consider the full interpersonal and cultural ecology within which the survivor lives, thinks, feels, behaves, and makes meaning. In describing clinical work with bereaved parents, Klass (2001) emphasizes the social and cultural dimensions of grief work:

> The consensus that seems to be emerging among scholars and clinicians is that the purpose or goal of grief is the construction of a durable biography, a narrative story that organizes and makes meaning of the survivor's life after the death as well as of the life of the person who died. The process by which this is achieved is active interaction within a community in which the death is recognized, the deceased person is mourned, and the continuing bond with the dead person is validated and shared. (p. 78)

The phenomenon of PTG has been examined in many different societies outside North America, including Germany, Spain, Japan, Australia, China, Israel, Turkey, and Kosovo (Weiss & Berger, 2010). Although PTG may show some similar features across cultures, a strong message in the cross-cultural work is that clinicians and counselors need to work within local norms and with respect to local narratives. Trauma may mean very different things in different cultures. Expectations regarding how one should respond to extremely negative life events, and the extent to which subsequent growth or benefit is even deemed to be possible in response to trauma, show substantial cross–cultural variation (Weiss & Berger, 2010). Some societies may consider certain traumas to be so bad or so debilitating that efforts to construct narratives of subsequent growth and redemption may be seen as doomed from the start, senseless, meaningless, and never-to-be believed or affirmed. In certain cultural contexts strong societal views on how one should process and talk about (or not talk about) things like suicide, pregnancy loss, stillbirth, and sexual assault will strongly influence the extent to which trauma victims may be able to adapt and grow from these experiences.

Within any given society, moreover, attitudes and stories about negative events change markedly over time. Outside the confessional and off the psychoanalytic couch, middle-class Americans in the 1950s and 1960s rarely narrated their traumatic events, if most sociological and cultural analyses are to be believed. However, in the past 30 years or so, these kinds of tellings have become more and more common—in 12-step programs, popular psychology books, memoirs and autobiographies, best-selling fiction, television shows, and the Internet (McAdams, 2006). Educated Americans today expect to hear stories about how personal trauma leads to growth. They find these stories much more compelling and coherent than they may have found them to be half a century ago, had they even had the rare opportunity, back then, to encounter just such an account.

As natural-born storytellers, human beings cannot help but make meaning out of their personal experiences. But every person makes meaning in a unique way, and within a specific social, cultural, and historical context. The context is key—the family members, friends, counselors, religious and cultural authorities, community resources, and prevailing cultural customs and institutions that ideally provide sustenance and support for the survivor. When trauma disrupts human lives and threatens to undermine cherished beliefs about self and world, people marshal all their powers to adapt, to move on, to change, and to grow. Amidst the horror and the heartbreak, it is of some comfort to know that there are many different paths people may take to find, and to live their way into, a better story for their lives, and that they need not take the journey alone.

REFERENCES

Adler, J. M., & Poulin, M. J. (2009). The political is personal: narrating 9/11 and psychological well-being. *Journal of Personality, 77*, 903–932.

Affleck, G., & Tennen, H. (1996). Construing benefits from adversity: adaptational significance and dispositional underpinnings. *Journal of Personality, 64*, 899–922.

Alon, N., & Omer, H. (2004). Demonic and tragic narratives in psychotherapy. In A. Lieblich, D. P. McAdams, & R. Josselson (Eds.), *Healing plots: The narrative bases of psychotherapy* (pp. 29–48). Washington, DC: APA Books.

Beike, D. R., & Crone, T. S. (2012). Autobiographical memory and personal meaning: stable versus flexible meanings of remembered life events. In P. T. P. Wong (Ed.), *The human quest for meaning* (2nd ed.) (pp. 315–334). New York: Routledge.

Bonanno, G. A. (2004). Grief, loss, and human resilience: have we underestimated the human capacity to thrive after extremely aversive events? *American Psychologist, 59*, 20–28.

Calhoun, L. G., & Tedeschi, R. G. (2001). Posttraumatic growth: the positive lessons of loss. In R. A. Neimeyer (Ed.), *Meaning reconstruction and the experience of loss* (pp. 157–172). Washington, DC: APA Books.

Davis, C. G. (2001). The tormented and the transformed: understanding responses to loss and trauma. In R. A. Neimeyer (Ed.), *Meaning reconstruction and the experience of loss* (pp. 137–155). Washington, DC: APA Books.

Davis, C. G., Nolen-Hoeksema, S., & Larson, J. (1998). Making sense of loss and benefitting from the experience: two construals of meaning. *Journal of Personality and Social Psychology, 75*, 561–574.

Etherington, K. (2008). *Trauma, drug misuse, and transforming identities: A life story approach.* London: Jessica Kingsley.

Frankl, V. (1959/1992). *Man's search for meaning* (4th ed.). Boston: Beacon Press.

Frazier, P. A. (2003). Perceived control and distress following sexual assault: a longitudinal test of a new model. *Journal of Personality and Social Psychology, 84*, 1257–1269.

Frazier, P. A., Tennen, H., Gavian, M., Park, C., Tomich, p., & Tashiro, T. (2009). Does self-reported posttraumatic growth reflect genuine positive change? *Psychological Science, 20*, 912–919.

Hammack, P. L. (2008). Narrative and the cultural psychology of identity. *Personality and Social Psychology Review, 12*, 222–247.

James, W. (1902/1958). *The varieties of religious experience.* New York: New American Library of World Literature.

Janoff-Bulman, R. (1992). *Shattered assumptions: Toward a new psychology of trauma.* New York: Free Press.

Joseph, S., & Linley, P. A. (2005). Positive adjustment to threatening events: an organismic valuing theory of growth through adversity. *Review of General Psychology, 9*, 262–280.

Kaminer, H., & Lavie, P. (1993). Sleep and dreams in well-adjusted and less adjusted holocaust survivors. In M. Stroebe, W. Stroebe, & R. O. Hansson (Eds.), *Handbook of bereavement: Theory, research, and intervention* (pp. 331–345). New York: Cambridge University Press.

King, L. A., & Hicks, J. A. (2007). What ever happened to "what might have been"? *American Psychologist, 62*, 625–636.

Klass, D. (2001). The inner representation of the dead child in the psychic and social narratives of bereaved parents. In R. A. Neimeyer (Ed.), *Meaning reconstruction and the experience of loss* (pp. 77–94). Washington, DC: APA Books.

Kushner, H. (1981). *When bad things happen to good people.* New York: Avon.

McAdams, D. P. (2006). *The redemptive self: Stories Americans live by.* New York: Oxford University Press.

McAdams, D. P., & Guo, J. (2015). Narrating the generative life. *Psychological Science, 26*, 475–483.

McAdams, D. P., & McLean, K. C. (2013). Narrative identity. *Current Directions in Psychological Science, 22*, 233–238.

Meichenbaum, D. (2006). Resilience and posttraumatic growth: a constructive narrative perspective. In L. G. Calhoun, & R. G. Tedeschi (Eds.), *Handbook of posttraumatic growth: Research and practice* (pp. 355–367). New York: Taylor & Francis.

Neimeyer, R. A. (2006). Re-storying loss: fostering growth in the posttraumatic narrative. In L. G. Calhoun, & R. G. Tedeschi (Eds.), *Handbook of posttraumatic growth: Research and practice* (pp. 68–80). New York: Taylor & Francis.

Ozer, E. J., Best, S. R., Lipsey, T. L., & Weiss, D. S. (2003). Predictors of posttraumatic stress disorder and symptoms in adults: a meta-analysis. *Psychological Bulletin, 129*, 52–73.

Pals, J. L. (2006). Constructing the "springboard effect": causal connections, self making, and growth within the life story. In D. P. McAdams, R. Josselson, & A. Lieblich (Eds.), *Identity and story: Creating self in narrative* (pp. 175–199). Washington, DC: APA Books.

Pals, J. L., & McAdams, D. P. (2004). The transformed self: a narrative understanding of post-traumatic growth. *Psychological Inquiry, 15,* 65–69.

Park, C. L. (2010). Making sense of the meaning literature: an integrative review of meaning making and its effects on adjustment to stressful events. *Psychological Bulletin, 136,* 257–301.

Park, C. L., Edmondson, D., Fenster, J. R., & Blank, T. O. (2008). Meaning making and psychological adjustment following cancer: the mediating roles of growth, life meaning, and restored just-world beliefs. *Journal of Consulting and Clinical Psychology, 76,* 863–875.

Sheikh, A. I. (2008). Posttraumatic growth in trauma survivors: implications for practice. *Counseling Psychology Quarterly, 21,* 85–97.

Silver, R. C., Boon, C., & Stones, M. H. (1983). Searching for meaning in misfortune: making sense of incest. *Journal of Social Issues, 39,* 81–102.

Silver, R. C., & Updegraff, J. A. (2013). Searching for and finding meaning following personal and collective traumas. In K. D. Markman, T. Proulx, & M. J. Lindberg (Eds.), *The psychology of meaning* (pp. 237–255). Washington, DC: APA Books.

Tedeschi, R. G., & Calhoun, L. G. (2004). Posttraumatic growth: the conceptual foundations and empirical evidence. *Psychological Inquiry, 15,* 1–18.

Weiss, T., & Berger, R. (Eds.). (2010). *Posttraumatic growth and culturally competent practice: Lessons learned from around the globe.* New York: Wiley.

CHAPTER 2

Meaning Violation and Restoration Following Trauma: Conceptual Overview and Clinical Implications

C.L. Park[1], M.C. Kennedy[2]
[1]University of Connecticut, Storrs, CT, United States; [2]Philadelphia University, Philadelphia, PA, United States

JANET

Janet was a 48-year-old married woman who presented with significant distress secondary to the death of her 18-year-old daughter in a car accident. Janet's medical history included a prior diagnosis of fibromyalgia, which resulted in significant physical impairment. At intake she required a cane for assistance with ambulation. She reported an inability to resume daily activities and admitted feeling deeply depressed and hopeless. Although suicide ideation was present, she had no plan or active intent. Janet agreed to seek treatment at the urging of her husband, who was concerned for her physical and mental health. After her daughter's accident, which had occurred 4 months prior, the physical symptoms associated with fibromyalgia became more pronounced and she was prescribed a high dose of prednisone to manage her pain. Her face and extremities were markedly swollen. She appeared in obvious physical, emotional, psychological, and spiritual distress.

Janet's most troublesome symptom early in therapy was her inability to stop the flood of images in her mind. Although not an eyewitness to the accident, she was well aware of its location and constructed a visual interpretation of the accident that repeated as an endless loop in her mind. She also imagined having dialogs with her daughter before she left the house in which she persuades her not to leave. These images prevented her from sleeping and from concentrating.

The early focus of counseling was on establishing a safe environment and attending to any questions or issues that impacted Janet's physical and

Reconstructing Meaning After Trauma
ISBN 978-0-12-803015-8
http://dx.doi.org/10.1016/B978-0-12-803015-8.00002-4

emotional safety. After safety was established, the counselor taught her relaxation techniques so that she would be able to calm her sympathetic nervous system initially in the office with the counselor and then later on her own. These techniques provided her with effective tools to deal with periodic eruptions of distress. As Janet began to feel more relaxed, she became better able to associate words with the disturbing images. The counselor advised her that she remained in control of the images of the accident and the parts that she felt safe to verbalize. This activity helped to reinforce her self-efficacy and sense of control. After attending to the specifics of her intrusive thoughts related to her daughter's accident, Janet was able to articulate her appraisal of the accident and how it violated her global meaning. Specifically, she believed God had abandoned her as evidenced in this freak single car accident, which occurred as a result of a rain-slicked road.

Despite the obvious role the weather played in the accident, Janet ruminated over the ways she believed she could have and should have prevented the accident. Before the accident, her daughter had informed her she was going out. Instead of persuading her otherwise, Janet advised her daughter to be careful. Given the resulting accident, Janet concluded that the responsibility for the event rested solely on her shoulders and her inability to prevent her daughter from leaving the safety of the house. She reported intense feelings of betrayal and anger. Her greatest sadness was losing her only daughter and all the unrealized dreams that died with her. She believed it was a universal wrong when children died before their parents.

THE MEANING MAKING MODEL

People navigate their lives through their global meaning systems. These meaning systems comprise people's fundamental beliefs—about themselves, the world, their place in the world, and their sense of meaning and purpose—as well as their unique hierarchies of goals and values. Global meaning systems inform people's understanding of themselves and their lives and direct their personal aims and projects and, through them, their general sense of well-being and life satisfaction (e.g., Emmons, 1999).

Global meaning influences appraisals of ordinary experiences as well as traumatic events. Meaning systems help people interpret and label the specific situations they encounter in life (e.g., appraisals of events' relevance, causality, threat, harm, loss, controllability), which then shape the emotional and behavioral consequences of these encounters (Folkman & Lazarus, 1980; Park, 2010). Situational meaning encompasses the meanings

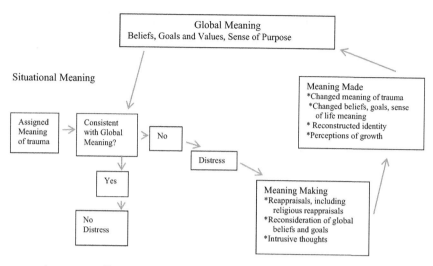

Figure 2.1 Meaning making model of trauma.

individuals assign to their experiences, the potential discrepancies between global and appraised meaning, the processes involved in reconciling those discrepancies (termed "meaning making"), and the changes resulting from these reconciliation processes (termed "meaning made"). Fig. 2.1 presents the meaning making model.

This chapter explicates the various aspects of global and situational meaning in the context of clinical work with trauma survivors. We draw upon the case of Janet throughout this chapter to illustrate the interplay of global and situational meanings in both the etiology of trauma-related distress and its resolution. We conclude with suggestions for applications of this model in clinical settings.

Global Meaning

Global meaning has three core elements—overarching beliefs, goals, and sense of meaning and purpose (Park & Folkman, 1997). As Janet's case illustrates, these elements inform individuals' meaning systems in profound ways, providing the frameworks through which they interpret, evaluate, and respond to their experiences.

Global beliefs. Global beliefs are widely encompassing assumptions about the self, others, and world, such as beliefs regarding the benevolence and fairness of the world, the nature of humanity, personal control, luck, randomness, and vulnerability, and how and why events occur (Janoff-Bulman, 1992; Koltko-Rivera, 2004). Global beliefs also include peoples' core views of themselves that form a sense of personal identity (Leary & Tangney, 2003). Every individual is unique in his or her specific constellations of beliefs, a result of a lifetime of exposure to direct and received experiences and one's continuous interpretation and reinterpretation of them (Christiansen, 2000; Leary & Tangney, 2003). For example, in Janet's case she believed that parents should outlive their children. In addition, she believed her main role as a parent was to protect and shield her daughter from harm. Her inability to do so resulted in significant guilt and self-judgment.

For many, spirituality, including their beliefs about God or of the Divine as loving and benevolent, wrathful, or distant, informs their core beliefs about the nature of people (e.g., inherent goodness, made in God's image, sinful human nature) and this world (e.g., the coming apocalypse, the illusory nature of reality), as well as, often, the next (e.g., heaven, reincarnation; Slattery & Park, 2011). Janet did not endorse a conventional religious perspective, but she did express a belief in transcendent energy and that life was somehow organized, ordered, and protected by this energy. It is interesting to note that when Janet expressed anger at the discrepancy between her spiritual beliefs and the accident she spoke of being "angry at God." The violation of her belief in a benevolent transcendent force set in motion a domino effect that toppled all other beliefs about the goodness of people and the inherent value of her life.

Although spirituality generally exerts positive influences on global beliefs, some spiritual beliefs can have negative content or exert negative influences on the believer as well. For example, some religious beliefs, such as those in an angry, uncaring, or punitive God, can have powerfully destructive implications for personal and social functioning in the context of stress or trauma (see Exline & Rose, 2013). In Janet's case she did not indicate a spiritual practice or community at intake. However, as is often the case, religious interpretations and spiritual implications are frequently manifest following trauma, even among those who profess to be a religious, and indeed, as we describe later, spiritual issues did play a role in her anguish.

Global goals. Global goals refer to people's motivation for living; choice of goals; standards for judging behavior, and basis for self-esteem; those high-level ideals, states, or objects that people work toward attaining or maintaining (Karoly, 1999; Klinger, 2012). Global goals commonly include relationships, work, health, wealth, knowledge, and achievement (Emmons, 2003). As a parent, Janet held goals for her daughter that included college, marriage, a career, and ultimately grandchildren. As an accomplished chef and gardener, Janet looked forward to entertaining her growing family and to caring for her grandchildren.

Sense of meaning and purpose. The emotional aspect of global meaning refers to the experience of a sense of meaning or purpose in life or as being connected to something greater than oneself (Klinger, 2012; Peterson, Park, & Seligman, 2005). Those who characterize their lives as high in meaning often believe that their lives are purposeful, comprehensible, and significant (Steger & Frazier, 2005). A strong sense of meaningfulness is manifested when one's global beliefs and goals are functioning well, allowing one to view his or her behaviors as consistent with core values and as representing progress toward desired future goals (McGregor & Little, 1998; Park, Edmondson, & Hale-Smith, 2013). Up until the accident, Janet reported her life had felt meaningful and her relationship with her daughter had been a major source of that meaning.

Situational Meaning

Situational meaning refers to how global meaning, within the context of a particular situation, influences one's reaction to that situation. Specifically, situational meaning includes the appraised meaning of the situation, detection of similarities and violations between that appraised meaning and global meaning, meaning making processes, and meaning made from the situation. In Janet's case, there was significant discrepancy among her global beliefs and goals and the meaning she attributed to the accident and the pervasive sense of loss it left in her life.

Appraised meaning of events. People appraise or assign meanings to situations that they encounter to understand their value and significance (Lazarus & Folkman, 1984). These appraised meanings are to some extent determined by the specific details of a given particular situation, but are largely informed by individuals' global meaning. Aspects of individuals' spiritual meaning systems can strongly influence their appraised meanings of specific situations. Despite her lack of reported spiritual involvement, Janet frequently mentioned her feeling that God had abandoned her, or that God had been derelict in His responsibility in not intervening to prevent the accident. Janet struggled to understand how an omniscient presence would allow such a tragedy. As a result, her sense of betrayal was deep and she often expressed rage at this "impotent" God.

Violations. After appraising the initial meaning of an event, individuals determine the extent to which that meaning is congruent with their global views of the world and themselves and their desires and goals. Myriad events are simply assimilated into global meaning, requiring little perceptual distortion or cognitive reworking. However, some events require accommodation to make sense of them, given their strong discrepancy with global meaning (Janoff-Bulman, 1992). The magnitude of the resultant distress corresponds to the extent to which global meaning has been violated (Janoff-Bulman, 1992; Steger, Owens, & Park, 2015). Janet believed that parents outlive their children. The violation of this deeply held belief resulted in crippling distress. Janet also held goals for her daughter and her future that included college, marriage, and children. The violation of these goals was particularly painful for Janet. She not only grieved the loss of her only child, but all the unrealized dreams that died with her.

Violations or discrepancies provide the impetus for initiating cognitive and emotional processing—"meaning making" efforts—to rebuild meaning systems in a manner that in some way accounts for the reality of the trauma. Meaning making involves efforts to understand and conceptualize stressors in ways that are more consistent with their global meaning and to incorporate that understanding into their larger system of global meaning through processes of assimilation and accommodation (Park & Folkman, 1997). Janet experienced significant and debilitating distress that manifested in emotional, behavioral, and physical symptoms. Attending first to the physical symptoms enabled the necessary process of meaning making to occur.

Meaning making. Mismatches between global and appraised meaning are distressing and people are often highly motivated to alleviate this distress (Greenberg, 1995; Janoff-Bulman, 1992; Joseph & Linley, 2005). When experiencing situations discrepant with their global meaning, people may respond in many different ways, including avoidance, distorting the experience, rumination, or seeking help to work through it, as Janet eventually opted to do. They may also attempt to directly solve or change the situation, often referred to as problem-focused coping (Aldwin, 2007); however, many of the most profound problems that create intense suffering cannot be directly solved and thus require meaning making to reduce and resolve violations.

Meaning making refers to attempts to resolve violations of global meaning by reaching a more acceptable appraisal of a distressing event to better incorporate it into one's existing global meaning system or changing one's global meaning to accommodate it (Park, 2010; Park & Folkman, 1997). Meaning making processes can include both automatic processes (such as intrusive thoughts and dreams) and more deliberate efforts (Park, 2010). Janet's frequent ruminations entailed what she should have said and done to prevent her daughter from leaving the home as well as asking larger questions of the universe, trying to understand how such a meaningless accident could occur.

The process of making meaning can be difficult and is often accompanied by increased anxiety, depression, rumination, and anger, as well as decrements in functioning. However, when people are able to make meaning of stressful situations—through constructing more benign situational meanings (e.g., I have been transformed and grown as a result of this trauma) and restoring or even creating more positive global meanings—they typically experience better adjustment to stressful events (Keesee, Currier, & Neimeyer, 2008). Janet frequently reported intrusive thoughts and images surrounding the accident. These eruptions occurred in every context of her life and without warning, leaving her feeling emotionally and physically "crippled." A key step in reducing her distress was to first promote relaxation techniques to encourage her body's natural tendency toward equilibrium. Over time, her subjective sense of diminished distress restored her self-worth and ability to regulate her emotions after which she and her counselor were able to process and rework her narrative of the event. To reinforce her sense of competency, the counselor affirmed her control over the images she wished to describe and the pace of her description. As counseling progressed, Janet would intersperse reflective comments into her unfolding narrative. These reflections served as the touchstones of her healing.

Meaning made. *Meaning made* refers to outcomes of these meaning making processes. These outcomes include changes in appraisals of a stressful event (e.g., coming to see it as less damaging or perhaps even fortuitous), changes in global meaning (e.g., changing one's identity to embrace the experience), and stress-related growth (e.g., experiencing increased appreciation for life, stronger connections with family and friends, or greater awareness of one's strengths; Park, 2010; Park, Edmondson, Fenster, & Blank, 2008). As illustrated in Fig. 2.1, making meaning of trauma can result in many different kinds of meaning made.

Successfully making meaning can reduce a sense of discrepancy between appraised and global meanings and restore a sense that the world is meaningful and life worthwhile. Over the course of time and in her process of retelling and writing her narrative of healing, Janet became aware of unique skills and strengths that before the accident were foreign to her. For example, she expressed a realization of her deep inner strength that enabled her to survive unspeakable loss; she became aware of her own ability to heal herself as evidenced in her diminished need for medications and her improved mobility. She drew energy from her heightened sense of strength and began to view life as purposeful. The experience of the tragedy initiated an intense search to find something redeemable. Janet was unwilling to view her daughter's death as arbitrary or meaningless but instead transformed her despair into a commitment to live fully and to appreciate each day as a gift.

CLINICAL IMPLICATIONS

The meaning making model, with variations, frequently serves as the basis of many clinical approaches to trauma (e.g., Aderka, Gillihan, McLean, & Foa, 2013; Morland, Hynes, Mackintosh, Resick, & Chard, 2011; Sloan, Marx, Bovin, Feinstein, & Gallagher, 2012), bereavement (e.g., Neimeyer Baldwin, & Gillies, 2006), and serious illness (Henry et al., 2010). Here, we briefly describe some of these applications and direct interested readers to resources from which they can learn more.

Assessment and Conceptualization

Conceptualizing a client presenting with trauma (or who may present with other concerns but also has a history of trauma) focuses on the discrepancies that the appraised meaning of the trauma represents for the client; that is, it is essential to assess the meaning which the client has assigned to the trauma, and how that meaning is congruent or discrepant with that client's global beliefs and goals as well as how it affects his or her sense of meaning in life. Using such an approach, it is important to attend to individuals' unique situational appraisals as well as their global meaning and goals. Tools for assessment of situational and global meaning have been described by Park and George (2013).

Interventions

Many widely used interventions for trauma survivors indirectly rely on meaning making notions. For example, cognitive processing therapy (CPT; Resick, Monson, & Chard, 2008) is a trauma-focused treatment that has consistently yielded benefits in improving posttraumatic stress disorder related to many different types of traumas (e.g., rape, childhood sexual abuse, military combat; see Cahill, Rothbaum, Resick, & Follette, 2009). In CPT the client processes and reprocesses the memory, including all of the client's appraised meanings of it, by first writing a detailed account of the trauma and then reading this account aloud in sessions with the therapist. The client also reviews the narrative at home over the initial weeks of treatment. CPT is consistent with a meaning making approach in its emphasis on the impact of trauma on aspects of a client's global meaning system and the necessary adjustments that must occur in the narrative account to adaptively reconcile situational meanings with the client's prior beliefs and goals.

In instances of severe distress, it is important to promote opportunities for the client to self-regulate and reduce distress so that they may engage in meaningful processing. In addition, CPT and other types of cognitive-behavioral therapies introduce activities that promote client self-efficacy early in the process, which positively impacts a client's sense of control over distressing symptoms. For example, in Janet's therapy, the counselor worked on first establishing safety and then introduced activities to promote self-efficacy.

Prolonged exposure (PE; Foa, Hembree, & Rothbaum, 2007) is a trauma-focused intervention that has received extensive empirical support (Powers Halpern, Ferenschak, Gillihan, & Foa, 2010). PE helps clients to revise their fear networks by activating these maladaptive structures within the therapeutic session while providing real-time information that is discrepant from the fear network. Through these exposures, PE indirectly addresses global beliefs commonly held by traumatized persons, such as that they lack control and the world is very dangerous. PE also involves repeatedly revisiting traumatic memories and engaging with painful emotional content both in sessions and listening to recordings of these exercises at home (i.e., imaginal exposure) and working through the emotional content and situational meanings of the trauma in open-ended discussions following imaginal exposure exercises.

In addition to the many excellent empirically validated treatments available to clinicians working with clients who have survived trauma, working from the meaning making perspective places a particular emphasis on the uniqueness of the inner world and understandings of experience that each specific client brings to the treatment. For example, in Janet's case, the counselor took the time to know and understand how Janet saw the world and her place in it, along the way learning that she was an accomplished chef, an avid gardener, a music aficionado, and a budding artist. In Janet's case, the counselor's understanding of Janet's meaning system allowed her to use her love of the natural world, her cooking, music, and drawing as ways for her to not only express her intense pain, but also craft her pathway to healing.

SUMMARY

The meaning making model provides a comprehensive framework for understanding how meaning is the basis of human functioning in everyday life, but is particularly relevant in the context of traumatic events. This model can be a helpful way to work with clients who have survived trauma. This perspective is consistent with the many existing and widely applied models of approaching trauma and complements them with a specific focus on the unique meanings of the particular client and his or her meaning system.

REFERENCES

Aderka, I. M., Gillihan, S. J., McLean, C. P., & Foa, E. B. (2013). The relationship between posttraumatic and depressive symptoms during prolonged exposure with and without cognitive restructuring for the treatment of posttraumatic stress disorder. *Journal of Consulting and Clinical Psychology, 81*, 375–383.

Aldwin, C. (2007). *Stress, coping, and development: An integrative perspective* (2nd ed.). New York: Guilford.

Cahill, S. P., Rothbaum, B. O., Resick, P. A., & Follette, V. M. (2009). Cognitive-behavioral therapy for adults. In E. B. Foa, T. M. Keane, M. J. Friedman, & J. A. Cohen (Eds.), *Effective treatments for PTSD: Practice guidelines from the society for traumatic stress studies* (2nd ed.) (pp. 139–222). New York, NY: Guilford.

Christiansen, C. (2000). Identity, personal projects and happiness: self construction in everyday action. *Journal of Occupational Science, 7*, 98–107.

Emmons, R. A. (1999). *The psychology of ultimate concerns*. New York: Oxford.

Emmons, R. A. (2003). Personal goals, life meaning, and virtue: wellsprings of a positive life. In C. L. M. Keyes, & J. Haidt (Eds.), *Flourishing: Positive psychology and the life well-lived* (pp. 105–128). Washington: American Psychological Association.

Exline, J. J., & Rose, E. D. (2013). Religious and spiritual struggles. In R. F. Paloutzian, & C. L. Park (Eds.), *Handbook of the psychology of religion and spirituality* (2nd ed.) (pp. 380–398). New York: Guilford.

Foa, E. B., Hembree, E. A., & Rothbaum, B. O. (2007). *Prolonged exposure therapy for PTSD: Emotional processing of traumatic experiences*. New York: Oxford.

Folkman, S., & Lazarus, R. S. (1980). An analysis of coping in a middle-aged community sample. *Journal of Health and Social Behavior, 21*, 219–239.

Greenberg, M. A. (1995). Cognitive processing of traumas: the role of intrusive thoughts and reappraisals. *Journal of Applied Social Psychology, 25*, 1262–1296.

Henry, M., Cohen, S. R., Lee, V., Sauthier, P., Provencher, D., Drouin, P., … Mayo, N. (2010). The Meaning-Making intervention (MMi) appears to increase meaning in life in advanced ovarian cancer: a randomized controlled pilot study. *Psycho-Oncology, 19*, 1340–1347.

Janoff-Bulman, R. (1992). *Shattered assumptions: Towards a new psychology of trauma*. New York: Free Press.

Joseph, S., & Linley, A. P. (2005). Positive adjustment to threatening events: an organismic valuing theory of growth through adversity. *Review of General Psychology, 9*, 262–280.

Karoly, P. (1999). A goal systems-self-regulatory perspective on personality, psychopathology, and change. *Review of General Psychology, 3*, 264–291.

Keesee, N. J., Currier, J. M., & Neimeyer, R. A. (2008). Predictors of grief following the death of one's child: the contribution of finding meaning. *Journal of Clinical Psychology, 64*, 1145–1163.

Klinger, E. (2012). The search for meaning in evolutionary goal-theory perspective and its clinical implications. In P. P. Wong (Ed.), *The human quest for meaning: Theories, research, and applications* (2nd ed.). New York: Routledge/Taylor & Francis Group.

Koltko-Rivera, M. E. (2004). The psychology of worldviews. *Review of General Psychology, 8*, 3–58.

Lazarus, R. S., & Folkman, S. (1984). *Stress, appraisal, and coping.* New York: Springer.

Leary, M. R., & Tangney, J. P. (2003). The self as an organizing construct in the behavioral sciences. In M. R. Leary, & J. P. Tangney (Eds.), *Handbook of self and identity* (pp. 3–14). New York: Guilford.

McGregor, I., & Little, B. R. (1998). Personal projects, happiness, and meaning: on doing well and being yourself. *Journal of Personality and Social Psychology, 74*, 494–512.

Morland, L. A., Hynes, A. K., Mackintosh, M. A., Resick, P. A., & Chard, K. M. (2011). Group cognitive processing therapy delivered to veterans via telehealth: a pilot cohort. *Journal of Traumatic Stress, 24*, 465–469.

Neimeyer, R. A., Baldwin, S. A., & Gillies, J. (2006). Continuing bonds and reconstructing meaning: mitigating complications in bereavement. *Death Studies, 30*, 715–738.

Park, C. L. (2010). Making sense of the meaning literature: an integrative review of meaning making and its effects on adjustment to stressful life events. *Psychological Bulletin, 136*, 257–301.

Park, C. L., Edmondson, D., Fenster, J. R., & Blank, T. O. (2008). Meaning making and psychological adjustment following cancer: the mediating roles of growth, life meaning, and restored just world beliefs. *Journal of Consulting and Clinical Psychology, 76*, 863–875.

Park, C. L., Edmondson, D., & Hale-Smith, A. (2013). Why religion? Meaning as motivation. In K. I. Pargament, J. J. Exline, J. Jones, & A. Mahoney (Eds.), *APA handbook of psychology, religion and spirituality* (pp. 157–171). Washington, DC: American Psychological Association.

Park, C. L., & Folkman, S. (1997). Meaning in the context of stress and coping. *Review of General Psychology, 1*, 115–144.

Park, C. L., & George, L. S. (2013). Assessing meaning and meaning making in the context of stressful life events: measurement tools and approaches. *Journal of Positive Psychology, 8*, 483–504.

Peterson, C., Park, N., & Seligman, M. E. P. (2005). Orientations to happiness and life satisfaction: the full life versus the empty life. *Journal of Happiness Studies, 6*, 25–41.

Powers, M. B., Halpern, J. M., Ferenschak, M. P., Gillihan, S. J., & Foa, E. B. (2010). A meta-analytic review of prolonged exposure for posttraumatic stress disorder. *Clinical Psychology Review, 30*, 635–641.

Resick, P. A., Monson, C. M., & Chard, K. M. (2008). *Cognitive processing therapy: Veteran/military version.* Washington, DC: Department of Veterans' Affairs.

Slattery, J. M., & Park, C. L. (2011). Meaning making and spiritually oriented interventions. In J. D. Aten, M. R. McMinn, & E. L. Worthington, Jr. (Eds.), *Spiritually oriented interventions for counseling and psychotherapy.* Washington, DC: American Psychological Association.

Sloan, D. M., Marx, B. P., Bovin, M. J., Feinstein, B. A., & Gallagher, M. W. (2012). Written exposure as an intervention for PTSD: a randomized clinical trial with motor vehicle accident survivors. *Behaviour Research and Therapy, 50*, 627–635.

Steger, M. F., & Frazier, P. (2005). Meaning in life: one link in the chain from religiousness to well-being. *Journal of Counseling Psychology, 52*, 574–582.

Steger, M. F., Owens, G. P., & Park, C. L. (2015). Violations of war: testing the meaning-making model among military veterans. *Journal of Clinical Psychology, 71*, 105–116.

CHAPTER 3

With the Fierce and Loving Embrace of Another Soul: Finding Connection and Meaning After the Profound Disconnection of Betrayal Trauma

P.J. Birrell[1], R.E. Bernstein[2], J.J. Freyd[2]
[1]Independent Practitioner, Eugene, OR, United States; [2]University of Oregon, Eugene, OR, United States

Amanda North[1] is a 50-year-old woman who has had problems with dissociation and depression most of her life. Her mother had died suddenly when she was 5 years old and her father remarried when she was eight. As an adult she was diagnosed with borderline personality disorder, anorexia nervosa, and major depression. She had been hospitalized for dissociation and an eating disorder and had had two failed attempts at psychotherapy wherein her therapists referred her on to someone new when she did not seem to be responding to their treatment. Amanda found her hospitalizations traumatic and destructive. She remembered meeting with one psychiatrist who had never made eye contact with her. She had been prescribed many psychiatric drugs and, when those failed, electroconvulsive therapy. Her therapists' referrals and the demeaning behavior of the hospital doctors and staff only reinforced her feeling that she was the problem and that everyone would be better off without her. The only thing that kept her going was her relationship with her daughter. When Amanda appeared in my office (senior author), she was hopeless and frightened. She did not know where to turn, but felt that somehow she had to find the truth of her life. She had very few early memories, and no conscious memories of trauma. It took much time to find out that Amanda's stepmother had not wanted children and had treated Amanda with contempt and anger. It took even longer than that to find that Amanda's father had molested her after her mother died, primarily because Amanda's memories of childhood were

---

[1] The client's name and details about her experience have been changed to protect her privacy. She has given her written permission to include this modified version of her story here.

Reconstructing Meaning After Trauma
ISBN 978-0-12-803015-8
http://dx.doi.org/10.1016/B978-0-12-803015-8.00003-6

sporadic and fragmented. Above all, she needed to believe that her father had taken care of her when she most needed it.

INTRODUCTION

To understand the reconstruction of meaning in the wake of trauma, it is first important to delineate both the nature of "trauma" and what it is that we mean by "meaning." In this chapter we shall examine the relational, contextual, and philosophical aspects of both trauma and meaning. Historically, psychology and psychiatry have emphasized the terror- and fear-inducing aspects of traumatic experiences on individuals, resulting in subsequent "pathology." Indeed, the inclusion of posttraumatic stress disorder (PTSD) in the Diagnostic and Statistical Manual of Mental Disorders, Third Edition (American Psychiatric Association, 1980) as a result of wartime experiences has put the emphasis on both fear [with many researchers and writers conceptualizing PTSD as a disorder of fear conditioning (Amstadter, Nugent, & Koenen, 2009; Fanselow & Ponnusamy, 2008; Milad et al., 2008; Peri, Ben-Shakhar, Orr, & Shalev, 2000)] and on individual "pathology"—symptoms of mental disorder that must be resolved so that the person can return to normal. Moreover, the effect of trauma on meaning has most often been conceptualized as the search of individual minds for new ideas to replace assumptions that have been shattered (Janoff-Bulman, 1992), following the emphasis in psychology of the cognitive revolution (see Miller, 2003).

In this chapter we will explore relational trauma, specifically Betrayal Trauma theory (BTT; Freyd, 1994, 1996), and relational meaning as that knowing that flows from relational connection.

PART I: TRAUMA AS BETRAYAL AND DISCONNECTION

As stated earlier, the field of traumatic stress has emphasized the importance of terror and life threat in predicting the psychological impact of trauma, and research has placed pathological fear at the core of posttraumatic stress (i.e., the "fear paradigm"; DePrince & Freyd, 2002). In contrast, BTT (Freyd, 1994, 1996) is a theory of psychological response to trauma that proposes that an individual's cognitive encoding of and response to trauma depends not only on the terror or fear of a specific event, but also on the event's social betrayal. More specifically, BTT "predicts that the degree to which a negative event represents a betrayal by a trusted, needed other will influence the way in which that event is processed and remembered" (Sivers, Schooler, & Freyd, 2002, p. 169). Indeed, we are social beings and depend on social connections for survival, nurturance, and meaning in our lives; it is no wonder that experiences that threaten our ability to trust and depend on others should be experienced in qualitatively different ways and should impact us in qualitatively different ways than noninterpersonal traumas. Betrayal, or relational trauma, by definition, involves loss and like all traumatic events "overwhelm[s] the ordinary systems of care that give people a sense of control, connection, and meaning" (Herman, 1997; p. 33). Although the losses implicated in relational trauma do not always involve maltreatment (as in the sudden death of a caregiver), in experiences of abuse, neglect, or abandonment, they may also represent violations of trust. When the latter is the case, betrayal trauma has occurred. Childhood abuse, infidelity, discrimination, and workplace or health place exploitation (the last example will be examined in the next section) are examples of betrayal trauma.

Although betrayal trauma refers to relational trauma independent of posttraumatic stress reactions (Freyd, 1996), and historically betrayal has not been included in diagnostic nosology, empirical evidence suggests that betrayal also plays an important role in the etiology of posttraumatic sequelae (e.g., DePrince et al., 2012; Gómez, Smith, & Freyd, 2014; Kelley, Weathers, Mason, & Pruneau, 2012). More specifically, the theory holds that the closer and more (apparently) necessary one's relationship is to the perpetrator(s), the greater the degree of betrayal involved. Although ordinarily, humans possess excellent cheater-detection capabilities (e.g., Cosmides & Tooby, 1992), under conditions where betrayal is strong, victims may experience "betrayal blindness" in which the betrayed person does not have conscious awareness of the betrayal.[2] This lack of awareness can manifest in several different ways, including an inability to recall the traumatic experience at all (i.e., amnesia), or being able to remember the events, but having a more benign (e.g., "it wasn't a big deal"), normalized (e.g., "that's how all families are"), or self-blaming (e.g., "it was my fault") interpretation of what transpired. Within this theoretical model, betrayal blindness serves the important and adaptive function of allowing individuals to maintain needed attachment relationships with their perpetrator(s) in situations where a full and conscious understanding of the betrayal could lead to withdraw or retaliatory behaviors that could threaten the persistence of the relationship. Consistent with this proposition, research has shown that even after controlling for age of abuse onset and abuse duration, the caregiver status of the

---

[2] John Bowlby (1980), the founder of Attachment theory, described a similar process as "defensive exclusion" or "defensive processing."

perpetrator predicts survivors' self-reported memory impairment (i.e., "I now remember basically what happened but I didn't always") for physical and sexual abuse experiences (Freyd, DePrince, & Zurbriggen, 2001).

BTT argues that over time (perhaps as a direct result of the trauma or perhaps by way of betrayal blindness) traumas high in betrayal will lead to dissociation, numbing, amnesia, and/or shame.[3] In support of the theory, a large and growing body of empirical work has shown that betrayal, and not fear, is strongly associated with dissociation (see DePrince & Freyd, 2007 for review). Betrayal has also been linked to shame, depression, chronic pain and gastrointestinal difficulties, inexplicable somatic symptoms (e.g., intermittent paralysis), and substance abuse, all of which are at least marginally related to the concept of dissociative unawareness (Delker & Freyd, 2014; Freyd, 1996; Goldsmith, Freyd, & DePrince, 2012; Martin, Cromer, DePrince, & Freyd, 2013; Platt & Freyd, 2012; Ross, 2005). Given that betrayal plays such an important role in influencing posttraumatic response, it follows that addressing experience(s) of relational rupture (e.g., betrayal) should be an important part of healing following betrayal trauma.

Betrayal Trauma and Interpersonal Connection. As outlined earlier, BTT posits that betrayal blindness is an adaptive human response to betrayal that allows individuals to maintain close relationships that they experience as necessary for their survival. Importantly, this posttraumatic response, although adaptive, is not without its drawbacks. Betrayal trauma has been linked to person-level difficulties in mental and physical health. On the level of interpersonal relationships, betrayal trauma and betrayal blindness have both been linked to various types of relationship difficulties. First, research has repeatedly shown that those who have experienced betrayal trauma are more likely to reexperience interpersonal trauma, a phenomenon known as revictimization (e.g., Gobin & Freyd, 2009). Researchers studying revictimization have posited that this pattern may be caused by the victim's diminished ability to perceive or drive to avoid risk. Gobin (2012) provided at least partial support for this hypothesis when she found that betrayal traumatization influences romantic partner preferences such that young adults who experienced high betrayal trauma in childhood rated loyalty as a less desirable trait in a potential romantic partner than those who did not, and

---

[3] The theory also holds that, consistent with a large body of research findings (e.g., Brett, 1996), traumas that are extremely frightening should lead to hypervigilance, hyperarousal, and/or anxiety. Like the causal pathway from betrayal to motivated unawareness, BTT maintains that the fear-to-hypervigilance causal pathway is also rooted in an evolutionary perspective and serves an adaptive function. More specifically, highly threatened individuals will be highly aware of signs of potential danger as a way to protect themselves against further harm.

those who experienced high betrayal trauma in both childhood and adulthood reported a higher tolerance for verbal aggression in a potential mate.

Second, studies of caregiver–infant relationships have shown that caregiver parental idealization [i.e., a form of betrayal blindness characterized by moderate to marked lack of unity between an individual's retrospective reports of (1) childhood experiences of unloving or abusive parenting and (2) how favorable or warm their relationships with their parent(s) had been (Hesse, 2008)] predicts avoidant infant–caregiver attachment[4] in the next generation. In one analysis, for example, infants' avoidance from their mothers during the reunion phases of the Strange Situation (Ainsworth, Blehar, Waters, & Wall, 1978) had a strong positive correlation with maternal idealization of their own mothers and fathers on George, Kaplan, and Main's (1985) Adult Attachment Interview (Hesse, 2008). A more recent study by the second author and colleagues found the same pattern of results when measuring parental idealization as discrepancies across two different retrospective self-report questionnaires on parental care received during childhood and betrayal trauma experienced during childhood (Bernstein, Laurent, Musser, Measelle, & Ablow, 2013). More specifically, results showed that while controlling for maternal demographics (i.e., education, ethnicity, and age) and both prenatal psychopathology and postnatal parental sensitivity to infant distress (both of which have been linked to child attachment outcomes; DeWolff & van IJzendoorn, 1997), parental idealization reported during pregnancy explained a unique 15.6% of the variance in secure versus avoidant caregiver–infant attachment at postnatal 18 months.

According to attachment theory, avoidant attachment is an adaptive defense against chronic caregiver rejection and aversion to physical closeness such that the infant has learned to inhibit his or her bids for proximity and suppress expressions of negative affect (which have been historically met with increased distance) as a way to reduce the chance of further rejection or abandonment (Ainsworth, Bell, & Stayton, 1971; Ainsworth et al., 1978; Cassidy, 1999; Koulomzin et al., 2002; Main & Stadtman, 1981; Sroufe, Egeland, Carlson, & Collins, 2005; Weinfield, Sroufe, Egeland, & Carlson, 1999). Given that betrayal blindness in the form of parental idealization predicts infant–caregiver attachment avoidance and that this avoidance is an adaptive response to caregiver rejection, it might be that betrayal blindness

---

[4] Infants are classified as having insecure-avoidant relationships with their primary caregivers when they avoid or ignore their caregiver when they are reunited after a brief separation during the Strange Situation—showing little overt indications of an emotional response. These infants often treat the stranger in the room in more or less the same way as their caregiver.

is part of what renders caregivers less able to respond sensitively to their infants in nonrejecting ways.

Of course, parents and caregivers are not the only perpetrators who are idealized by victims of betrayal trauma. Adults who are in the midst of a violent relationship with a romantic partner, especially those who are most reluctant to leave their abusive romantic partner (due to threat of increased violence, financial dependence, etc.; Freyd, 1996), are also likely to idealize their abusers (Douglas, 1987; Dutton & Painter, 1981, 1993). In both of these relationships, victims of betrayal idealize their perpetrators and do not blame them for any wrongdoings (placing the blame instead on themselves or someone external to the relationship) so as to preserve the relationship between themselves and their abuser. In other words, the meaning they construct regarding the relationship as a whole, and regarding remembered abuse, neglect, rejection, or other unloving behavior more specifically, is designed to be compatible with maintaining the relationship.

Amanda, who was introduced at the beginning of this chapter and who had clearly had been betrayed in her life, shared multiple indications of parental idealization. The early death of her mother was never explained to her and her fragmentary memories of her mother's funeral were very disturbing to her. She grew up thinking that somehow she had been the cause of her mother's death. Consciously she saw her father as her savior and hero. She had no conscious knowledge of him molesting her. As BTT would predict, Amanda split off memories of the nightly visits to protect her relationship with her father. Conscious knowledge of his betrayal would have left her with no parent and no place to go. When her father remarried, her stepmother was rigid and constantly complained about Amanda to friends in Amanda's presence. She did not know how to nurture a child. As an example, Amanda was terrified of thunderstorms and was made to be alone in her room during the frequent and violent midwest thunderstorms. Amanda remembered these storms as some of the most terrifying moments of her life and has remained terrified of them.

PART II: INSTITUTIONAL BETRAYAL

Although early formulations of betrayal trauma theory (e.g., Freyd, 1996) encompassed the possibility of betrayal by social groups (e.g., the Holocaust), the empirical research in betrayal trauma began with a focus on emotional, physical, and sexual abuse perpetrated by one individual against another individual (e.g., abuse within a parent–child relationship, domestic violence between romantic partners, assault or harassment between an employer and employee). In recent years the field has expanded to explore betrayal trauma as it occurs between individuals and institutions (e.g., Smith & Freyd, 2013), which often elicit similar trust and dependency from their members as is the case within interpersonal relationships (Baker, McNeil, & Siryk, 1985; Cardador, Dane, & Pratt, 2011; Somers, 2010; Tremblay, 2010). As with trusted interpersonal relationships, institutions are frequently expected to be safe (Platt, Barton, & Freyd, 2009; Tremblay, 2010) and in some cases, may be quite literally depended on for survival (e.g., as is true with Medicaid for low-income families and the military for soldiers; Suris, Lind, Kashner, & Borman, 2007). Within this emerging area, "institutional betrayal" refers to an institution's perpetration of mistreatment (e.g., a nursing home administration's active approval of involuntary sterilization of intellectually disabled residents) or their failure (whether by commission or omission) to prevent or respond supportively following mistreatment within the institution (e.g., a sexual assault at a military base, a case of medical malpractice at a hospital, a college campus' unlawful release of private medical records).

In one study of undergraduate women, Smith and Freyd (2013) found that nearly half of the women who had had at least one unwanted sexual experience while in college reported at least some degree of additional institutional betrayal by their university related to the assault (e.g., creating an environment where these experiences seemed more likely, making it difficult to report these experiences). Moreover, the women who reported experiencing institutional betrayal surrounding their unwanted sexual experience reported increased levels of anxiety, trauma-specific sexual symptoms, dissociation, and problematic sexual functioning, indicating that institutions have the power to cause additional harm to survivors of interpersonal trauma.

Some of Amanda's experiences with the mental health system are examples of institutional betrayal trauma. Amanda was distressed, fragmented, desperate, and despairing when she went for help. She was engaging in self-harming behaviors that both provided her some relief and frightened her badly. She did not understand those behaviors, nor did she understand her refusal to eat or the voices she sometimes heard. Rather than helping her understand her reactions or validate her experiences, feelings, and coping strengths, Amanda was pathologized. Amanda's voices and her self-harming behaviors (cutting and burning) were conceptualized as "symptoms" of her mental illness and she was put on behavioral programs and psychiatric drugs to control them. She was then further humiliated when two therapists to whom she had become attached communicated that they could no longer see her. Without clear early memories the voices that Amanda sometimes heard and the pictures that she saw in her head made no sense. The mental health system failed to treat Amanda with respect and conveyed to her a perspective that undermined her basic dignity and well-being. Amanda was indeed lost and the world around her was without meaning.

PART III: MEANING, AUTHENTICITY, AND CONNECTION

There has been much research and interest in the concept of meaning in psychology, and specifically in finding meaning after traumatic experiences (for a review, see Park, 2010). In most of this research, the individual anxiety and fear dimension of trauma, rather than the social betrayal dimension, has been assumed to be central. Meaning has been defined as a "mental representation of possible relationships among things, events, and relationships. Thus, meaning *connects* things" (Baumeister, 1991, p. 15). The "things" that get connected have most often been assumed to be global and situational appraisals, shattered assumptions (Janoff-Bulman, 1992), and discrepancies between the worldview before the trauma and after the trauma (Park, 2010). The meaning making model postulates that recovering from a stressful event involves reducing the discrepancy between its appraised meaning and global beliefs and goals (Joseph & Linley, 2005). Meaning making from this traditional perspective thus refers to the processes in which people engage to reduce this discrepancy. In other words, after a trauma that shatters our outer and inner worlds, we ask why and attempt to bring together our global and situational appraisals and restore our inner sense of mental meaning—thoughts and appraisals come together and an inner order is restored.

The betrayal aspect of trauma alerts us to a different domain of meaning. Betrayal trauma, and especially early developmental trauma, shatters not only our assumptions (since assumptions have not been made) but also our needed emotional bonds and we are thrown into inner chaos beyond conscious thought (Stolorow, 2015). Stolorow (2015) refers to this state as disorganized self-states that result from early emotional trauma:

> …[E]motional trauma is an experience of unendurable emotional pain and, further, that the unbearability of emotional suffering cannot be explained solely, or even primarily, on the basis of the intensity of the painful feelings evoked by an injurious event. Painful emotional states become unbearable when they cannot find a context of emotional understanding—what I came to call a relational home—in

which they can be shared and held. Severe emotional pain that has to be experienced alone becomes lastingly traumatic and usually succumbs to some form of emotional numbing. In contrast, painful feelings that are held in a context of human understanding can gradually become more bearable.

p. 124–125.

The self-state referred to by Stolorow in this quote bears an uncanny resemblance to what Miller calls "Condemned isolation" (Miller, 1988), or the experience of isolation and aloneness that leaves one feeling shut out of the human community. One feels alone, immobilized regarding reconnection, and at fault for this state. There is no "relational home" (Stolorow, 2015) in which to process these fragments. In addition, there is a severe constriction of emotional experience in which parts of the child's emotional world are sacrificed to keep the needed tie, another consequence of betrayal in early childhood.

This condemned isolation view, as with the quote by Stolorow, is very different from the emotional processing referred to in most current research about "meaning." However, Rachman (1980) described *emotional processing*, referring to "a process whereby emotional disturbances are absorbed, and decline to the extent that other experiences and behaviour can proceed without disruption" (Rachman, 2001, p. 165). Whether it is this emotional processing or a combined emotion–cognitive processing (Hayes, Laurenceau, Feldman, Strauss, & Cardaciotto, 2007) that occurs, the meaning making that must follow after early betrayal goes far beyond this to the construction or reconstruction of self, a process that cannot be done without restoring social bonds (Stolorow, 2013).

Judith Herman (1992) puts it this way: "…under conditions of chronic childhood abuse, fragmentation becomes the central principle of personality organization. Fragmentation in consciousness prevents the ordinary integration of knowledge, memory, emotional states, and bodily experience. Fragmentation in the inner representations of the self prevents the integrations of identity. Fragmentation in the inner representations of others prevents the development of a reliable sense of independence within connection" (p. 107). In other words, those traumas that involve betrayal cut us off from connection with others and even a basic sense of "being" within ourselves.

Meaning for human beings, then, is not just about cognitive appraisal of "things" or the way the world works: it is also about the meaning of relationships in one's life. At the end of one's life it is very likely that the meaning of life will be understood as fundamentally about relationships. Meaning comes from a sense of belonging—"To Belong is to Matter" (Lambert et al., 2013). Betrayal shatters not only our assumptions about the world and illusions of everyday life. But it also exposes us to a universe that is random and unpredictable and in which no safety or continuity of being can be assured. Trauma thereby exposes "the unbearable embeddedness of being" (Stolorow & Atwood, 1992, p. 22), and highlights the trauma survivor's lack of belonging and embeddedness.

For those who have suffered betrayal, making meaning after trauma, then, is connection both within themselves and connection with the wider community from which they have been cut off. This connection is not from the cognitive or even emotional putting together of existing thoughts, emotions, and assumptions, but a coalescence of unheld affect and experience finding each other in a relational home. If authentic connection and the reparation of disconnections are the source of healing and growth, whereas chronic disconnections are the primary source of suffering, then every moment in therapy potentially becomes an important moment of connection and of emotional dwelling (Birrell, 2006; Miller & Stiver, 1994, 1997; Stolorow, 2015). Birrell (2011) has extended this to the idea of a relational ethic, arguing that there are three dimensions that must be addressed to come to a true relational ethic: power, compassion, and the ability to be with uncertainty in relational space. The ethics of relational engagement consists of full presence, not only to the other but also to the self and to the space between.

This can be related to the idea of authenticity in both existential thought and relational cultural theory (Donaghy, 2002; Miller et al., 1999). In relational cultural therapy, authenticity is defined as "a person's ongoing ability to represent... [themselves] ...in relationships more fully" (Miller et al., 1999, p. 5). It also means being present with one's whole being with the ability to listen not only to verbal and nonverbal communications, but also to the space between (Bergum & Dossetor, 2005; Winnicott, 1971). It is only in our own authenticity that we can allow the other to be truly authentic (Miller et al., 1999). In this process, the goal is connection, not repair; and meaning results from this connection. The connection itself is the healing agent, as those who have experienced betrayal trauma have suffered fundamental disconnection.

Ethical approaches to dealing with those who have suffered deep betrayals require an ethic of "meeting each other as 'brothers and sisters in the same dark night' (Vogel, 1994, p. 97)," deeply connected with one another in virtue of our common finitude. Thus, although the possibility of emotional trauma is ever present, so too is the possibility of forming bonds of deep emotional attunement within which devastating emotional pain can be held, rendered more tolerable, and, hopefully, eventually integrated. Our existential kinship-in-the-same-darkness is the condition for the possibility both of the profound contextuality of emotional trauma and of the mutative power of human understanding (Stolorow, 2015, p. 136). These ways of being in an ethical relation with those most deeply betrayed can lead us to uncertainty in our epistemology, in our relationships, and in our concept of what it means to be a self. They lead us from the realm of justice and rights to that of love and compassion (Birrell, 2006).

Amanda's initial desperation and despair came from a lack of meaning and a lack of connection. Her behaviors and "symptoms" made no sense to her because they were removed from the context of her life. She was disconnected from herself and from others. Since the time of her mother's death it had not been safe to know the truth of her own life, so she had constructed a self that was acceptable to others, but lacked cohesiveness and meaning. Amanda was able to discover some of the truths of her life in a relationship that was real, authentic, and accepting. In this authentic connection, Amanda was able to remember the scene at the lake during a thunderstorm when her father had first molested her. She was able to recognize her internal voices as those of her stepmother who had shamed her for most of her childhood. She was able to make meaning of all the "symptoms" that had plagued her through the years as messages and reminders of wholeness. She was able to recover meaning that was initially lost by betrayal. Most of all, she was able to recover meaning in the wholeness and in being held in a relational home. The meaning that she found was not the putting together of cognitive constructs after terror, but from finding a place in a relational world after profound betrayal.

Perhaps meaning, as we are speaking about here, is better expressed in poetry rather than mental representation. Amanda wrote this poem at the end of her treatment.[5]

Coming Back

What is it to come back?
Is it a return to a source deep and soulful
Or a destination finally reached.
Perhaps it is a clearing of the heart and mind
Allowing the true self to emerge.

---

[5] Amanda has given written permission to use this poem.

Is it a return to previously held convictions
Or to discover our genuine beliefs.
Perhaps it is a rebirth of Spirit opening itself within
Our being now awash with the light of purpose.
Coming back is to step forward from the depths of the cavernous past
To explore and expose terrors pocketed away so long ago.
Cleansing heart mind and soul as they are brought into light
With the fierce and loving embrace of another soul.

REFERENCES

Ainsworth, M. D. S., Bell, S. M., & Stayton, D. (1971). Individual differences in strange situation behavior of one-year-olds. In H. R. Schaffer (Ed.), *The origins of human social relations* (pp. 17–57). London: Academic Press.
Ainsworth, M. D. S., Blehar, M., Waters, E., & Wall, S. (1978). *Patterns of attachment*. Hillsdale, NJ: Erlbaum.
American Psychiatric Association. (1980). *Diagnostic and statistical manual of mental disorders* (3rd ed.). Washington, DC: Author.
Amstadter, A. B., Nugent, N. R., & Koenen, K. C. (2009). Genetics of PTSD: fear conditioning as a model for future research. *Psychiatric Annals, 39*, 358–367.
Baker, R., McNeil, O., & Siryk, B. (1985). Expectation and reality in freshman adjustment to college. *Journal of Counseling Psychology, 32*, 94–103. http://dx.doi.org/10.1037/0022-0167.32.1.94.
Baumeister, R. F. (1991). *Meanings in life*. New York, NY: Guilford.
Bergum, V., & Dossetor, J. (2005). *Relational ethics: The full meaning of respect*. Hagerstown, MD: University Publishing Group.
Bernstein, R. E., Laurent, H. K., Musser, E. D., Measelle, J. R., & Ablow, J. C. (2013). In an idealized world: can discrepancies across self-reported parental care and betrayal trauma during childhood predict infant attachment avoidance in the next generation? *Journal of Trauma & Dissociation, 14*, 529–545. http://dx.doi.org/10.1080/15299732.2013.773476.
Birrell, P. J. (2006). An ethic of possibility: relationship, risk, and presence. *Ethics & Behavior, 16*, 95–115.
Birrell, P. (2011). *Ethics and power: Navigating mutuality in therapeutic relationships*. Wellesley Centers for Women Work in Progress Series, #108. Wellesley, MA: Wellesley Centers for Women.
Bowlby, J. (1980). Attachment and loss. *Loss, sadness and depression* (Vol. 3). New York: Basic Books.
Brett, E. A. (1996). The classification of posttraumatic stress disorder. In B. A. van der Kolk, A. C. McFarlane, & L. Weisaeth (Eds.), *Traumatic stress: The effects of overwhelming experience on mind, body, and society* (pp. 117–128). New York: Guilford Press.
Cardador, M., Dane, E., & Pratt, M. (2011). Linking calling orientations to organizational attachment via organizational instrumentality. *Journal of Vocational Behavior, 79*, 367–378. http://dx.doi.org/10.1016/j.jvb.2011.03.009.
Cassidy, J. (1999). The nature of the child's ties. In J. Cassidy, & P. Shaver (Eds.), *Handbook of attachment: Theory, research, and clinical applications* (pp. 3–20). New York: Guilford Press.
Cosmides, L., & Tooby, J. (1992). Cognitive adaptations for social exchange. In J. H. Barkow, L. Cosmides, & J. Tooby (Eds.), *The adapted mind: Evolutionary psychology and the generation of culture* (pp. 163–228). New York: Oxford University Press.
Delker, B. C., & Freyd, J. J. (2014). From betrayal to the bottle: investigating possible pathways from trauma to problematic substance use. *Journal of Traumatic Stress, 27*, 576–584.

DePrince, A. P., Brown, L. S., Cheit, R. E., Freyd, J. J., Gold, S. N., Pezdek, K., ... Quina, K. (2012). Motivated forgetting and misremembering: perspectives from betrayal trauma theory. In R. F. Belli (Ed.), *True and false recovered memories: toward a reconciliation of the debate (Nebraska symposium on motivation 58)* (pp. 193–243). New York: Springer.

DePrince, A. P., & Freyd, J. J. (2002). The harm of trauma: pathological fear, shattered assumptions, or betrayal? In J. Kauffman (Ed.), *Loss of the assumptive world: A theory of traumatic loss* (pp. 71–82). New York: Brunner-Routledge.

DePrince, A. P., & Freyd, J. J. (2007). Trauma-induced dissociation. In M. J. Friedman, T. M. Keane, & P. A. Resick (Eds.), *Handbook of PTSD: Science & practice* (pp. 135–150). New York: Guilford Press.

DeWolff, M. S., & van IJzendoorn, M. H. (1997). Sensitivity and attachment: a meta-analysis on parental antecedents of infant attachment. *Child Development, 68*, 571–591.

Donaghy, M. (2002). Authenticity: a goal for therapy? *Practical Philosophy*, 40–45.

Douglas, M. A. (1987). The battered women syndrome. In D. J. Sonkin (Ed.), *Domestic violence on trial: Psychological and legal dimensions of family violence* (pp. 39–54). New York: Springer.

Dutton, D. G., & Painter, S. L. (1981). Traumatic bonding: the development of emotional attachments in battered women and other relationships of intermittent abuse. *Victimology, 6*, 139–155.

Dutton, D. G., & Painter, S. L. (1993). The battered woman syndrome: effects of severity and intermittency of abuse. *American Journal of Orthopsychiatry, 63*, 614–622.

Fanselow, M. S., & Ponnusamy, R. (2008). The use of conditioning tasks to model fear and anxiety. In R. J. Blanchard, D. C. Banchard, G. Griebel, & D. J. Nutt (Eds.), *Handbook of anxiety and fear* (pp. 29–48). Países Bajos: Elsevier.

Freyd, J. J. (1994). Betrayal trauma: traumatic amnesia as an adaptive response to childhood abuse. *Ethics & Behavior, 4*, 307–329.

Freyd, J. J. (1996). The science of memory: apply with caution. *Traumatic Stress Points, 10*(1), 8.

Freyd, J. J., DePrince, A. P., & Zurbriggen, E. L. (2001). Self-reported memory for abuse depends upon victim-perpetrator relationship. *Journal of Trauma & Dissociation, 2*, 5–17.

George, C., Kaplan, N., & Main, M. (1985). *Adult attachment Interview. Unpublished protocol.* Berkeley: University of California.

Gobin, R. L. (2012). Partner preferences among survivors of betrayal trauma. *Journal of Trauma & Dissociation, 13*, 152–174.

Gobin, R. L., & Freyd, J. J. (2009). Betrayal and revictimization: preliminary findings. *Psychological Trauma: Theory, Research, Practice, and Policy, 1*, 242–257.

Goldsmith, R., Freyd, J. J., & DePrince, A. P. (2012). Betrayal trauma: associations with psychological and physical symptoms in young adults. *Journal of Interpersonal Violence, 27*, 547–567.

Gómez, J. M., Smith, C. P., & Freyd, J. J. (2014). Zwischenmenschlicher und institutioneller verrat [interpersonal and institutional betrayal]. In R. Vogt (Ed.), *Verleumdung und Verrat: Dissoziative Störungen bei schwer traumatisierten Menschen als Folge von Vertrauensbrüchen* (pp. 82–90). Roland, Germany: Asanger Verlag.

Hayes, A. M., Laurenceau, J., Feldman, G., Strauss, J. L., & Cardaciotto, L. (2007). Change is not always linear: the study of nonlinear and discontinuous patterns of change in psychotherapy. *Clinical Psychology Review, 27*, 715–723.

Herman, J. (1992). Complex PTSD: a syndrome in survivors of prolonged and repeated trauma. *Journal of Traumatic Stress, 5*, 377–391. http://dx.doi.org/10.1002/jts.2490050305.

Herman, J. L. (1997). *Trauma and recovery.* New York: Basic Books.

Hesse, E. (2008). The Adult Attachment Interview: protocol, method of analysis, and empirical studies. In J. Cassidy, & P. R. Shaver (Eds.), *Handbook of attachment: Theory, research, and clinical applications* (2nd ed.) (pp. 552–598). New York, NY: Guilford Press.

Janoff-Bulman, R. (1992). *Shattered assumptions: Towards a new psychology of trauma*. New York: Free Press.

Joseph, S., & Linley, P. A. (2005). Positive adjustment to threatening events: an organismic valuing theory of growth through adversity. *Review of General Psychology*, 262–280.

Kelley, L. P., Weathers, F. W., Mason, E. A., & Pruneau, G. M. (2012). Association of life threat and betrayal with posttraumatic stress disorder symptom severity. *Journal of Traumatic Stress*, *25*, 408–415. http://dx.doi.org/10.1002/jts.21727.

Koulomzin, M., Beebe, B., Anderson, S., Jaffe, J., Feldstein, S., & Crown, C. (2002). Infant gaze, head, face, and self-touch at four months differentiate secure vs. avoidant attachment at one year: a microanalytic approach. *Attachment and Human Development*, *4*, 3–24.

Lambert, N. M., Stillman, T. F., Hicks, J. A., Baumeister, R. F., Gamble, S., & Fincham, F. D. (2013). To belong is to matter: sense of belonging enhances meaning in life. *Personality and Social Psychology Bulletin*, 39, 1418–1427.

Main, M., & Stadtman, J. (1981). Infant response to rejection of physical contact by the mother: aggression, avoidance and conflict. *Journal of the American Academy of Child Psychiatry*, *20*, 2992–3007.

Martin, C. G., Cromer, L. D., DePrince, A. P., & Freyd, J. J. (2013). The role of cumulative trauma, betrayal, and appraisals in understanding trauma symptomatology. *Psychological Trauma: Theory, Research, Practice, and Policy*, *5*, 110–118.

Milad, M. R., Orr, S. P., Lasko, N. B., Chang, Y., Rauch, S. L., & Pitman, R. K. (2008). Presence and acquired origin of reduced recall for fear extinction in PTSD: results of a twin study. *Journal of Psychiatric Research*, *42*, 515–520.

Miller, G. A. (2003). The cognitive revolution: a historical perspective. *TRENDS in Cognitive Sciences*, 7, 141–144.

Miller, J. B. (1988). *Connections, disconnections, and violations. Work in Progress, No. 33.* Wellesley, MA: Stone Center Working Paper Series.

Miller, J. B., Jordan, J. V., Stiver, I. P., Walker, M., Surrey, J., & Eldridge, N. S. (1999). *Therapists' authenticity (work in progress no. 82)*. Wellesley, MA: Stone Center Working Paper Series.

Miller, J. B., & Stiver, I. P. (1994). *Movement in therapy: Honoring the strategies of disconnection*. Wellesley, MA: The Stone Center.

Miller, J. B., & Stiver, I. P. (1997). *The healing connection*. Boston: Beacon Press.

Park, C. L. (2010). Making sense of the meaning literature: an integrative review of meaning making and its effects on adjustment to stressful life events. *Psychology Bulletin*, *136*, 257–301.

Peri, T., Ben-Shakhar, G., Orr, S. P., & Shalev, A. Y. (2000). Psychophysiologic assessment of aversive conditioning in posttraumatic stress disorder. *Biological Psychiatry*, *47*, 512–519.

Platt, M., Barton, J., & Freyd, J. J. (2009). A betrayal trauma perspective on domestic violence. In E. Stark, & E. S. Buzawa (Eds.), *Violence against women in families and relationships* (Vol. 1) (pp. 185–207). Westport, CT: Greenwood Press.

Platt, M., & Freyd, J. J. (2012). Trauma and negative underlying assumptions in feelings of shame: an exploratory study. *Psychological Trauma: Theory, Research, Practice, and Policy*, *4*, 370–378.

Rachman, S. (1980). Emotional processing. *Behaviour Research and Therapy*, *18*, 51–60.

Rachman, S. (2001). Emotional processing, with special reference to post-traumatic stress disorder. *International Review of Psychiatry*, *13*, 164–171.

Ross, C. (2005). Long term effects of child sexual abuse: childhood sexual abuse and psychosomatic symptoms in irritable bowel syndrome. *Journal of Child Sexual Abuse: Research, Treatment, & Program Innovations for Victims, Survivors, & Offenders*, *14*, 27–38. http://dx.doi.org/10.1300/J070v14n0.

Sivers, H., Schooler, J., & Freyd, J. J. (2002). Recovered memories. In V. S. Ramachandran (Ed.), *Encyclopedia of the human Brain* (Vol. 4) (pp. 169–184). San Diego, California and London: Academic Press.

Smith, C. P., & Freyd, J. J. (2013). Dangerous safe havens: institutional betrayal exacerbates sexual trauma. *Journal of Traumatic Stress, 26*, 119–124.

Somers, M. (2010). Patterns of attachment to organizations: commitment profiles and work outcomes. *Journal of Occupational & Organizational Psychology, 83*, 443–453. http://dx.doi.org/10.1348/096317909x424060.

Sroufe, L. A., Egeland, B., Carlson, E. A., & Collins, W. A. (2005). *The development of the person: The Minnesota Study of Risk and Adaptation from Birth to Adulthood.* New York: Guilford Press.

Stolorow, R. D. (2013). Intersubjective-systems theory: a phenomenological-contextualist psychoanalytic perspective. *Psychoanalytic Dialogues, 23*, 383–389.

Stolorow, R. D. (2015). A phenomenological-contextual, existential, and ethical perspective on emotional trauma. *Psychoanalytic Review, 102*, 123–138.

Stolorow, R. D., & Atwood, G. E. (1992). *Contexts of being: The intersubjective foundations of psychological life.* Hillsdale, NJ: Analytic Press.

Suris, A., Lind, L., Kashner, M., & Borman, P. D. (2007). Mental health, quality of life, and health functioning in women veterans: differential outcomes associated with military and civilian sexual assault. *Journal of Interpersonal Violence, 22*, 179–197. http://dx.doi.org/10.1177/0886260506295347.

Tremblay, M. (2010). Fairness perceptions and trust as mediators on the relationship between leadership style, unit commitment, and turnover intentions of Canadian forces personnel. *Military Psychology, 22*, 510–523. http://dx.doi.org/10.1080/08995605.2010.513271.

Vogel, L. (1994). *The fragile "we": Ethical implications of Heidegger's being and time.* Evanston, Ill: Northwestern University Press.

Weinfield, N. S., Sroufe, L. A., Egeland, B., & Carlson, E. (1999). The nature of individual differences in infant-caregiver attachment. In J. Cassidy & P. Shaver (Eds.), *Handbook of Attachment: Theory, research, and clinical application* (pp. 68–88). New York: Guilford Press.

Winnicott, D. W. (1971). *Playing and reality.* UK: Tavistock Publications.

PART 2

Mechanisms of Meaning Loss and Restoration

CHAPTER 4

Gender and Meaning Making: The Experiences of Individuals With Cancer

M.A. Keitel, K. Lipari, H. Wertz
Fordham University, New York, NY, United States

GENDER AND MEANING MAKING: THE EXPERIENCES OF INDIVIDUALS WITH CANCER

Antonio, a 46-year-old Mexican-born man living in Texas, underwent laparoscopic radical prostatectomy for prostate cancer approximately a year ago. His diagnosis was delayed by a cultural belief that one should only see a doctor when symptoms emerge. Antonio's reluctance to see a doctor was only exacerbated by the fact that a common screening method for prostate cancer is a digital rectal examination that he considered "unmanly," as it requires the doctor to insert a finger into the rectum. He has always been athletic and relatively healthy, so the cancer diagnosis was particularly shocking. Antonio grew up in a culture that expected men to be stoic and strong; despite this, he openly shares many of his feelings with his wife of 25 years who he considers his primary support. Antonio does not cry in front of his wife or his two teen-aged children, however, and expends much energy keeping his fears to himself. Antonio has friends with whom he enjoys sports and other recreational activities but he does not confide in any of them. He also is influenced by the cultural construct of *caballerismo* (i.e., the man as the respected protector of and provider for the family). His identity as "the family protector" is seriously challenged by his cancer diagnosis and treatment. Antonio thinks if he communicates a positive and hopeful attitude, the experience will be easier for him and his family. Before his surgery, Antonio worked over 70 h per week as a manager in a close friend's restaurant. He was out of work for 6 weeks following the procedure and was ambivalent about returning because he did not yet have full bladder control. Antonio wanted to appear strong, healthy, and in control to ensure that his coworkers treated him as they always had. He was ready to move on from

Reconstructing Meaning After Trauma
ISBN 978-0-12-803015-8
http://dx.doi.org/10.1016/B978-0-12-803015-8.00004-8

the illness and thought no one was interested in hearing his problems. The way he saw it, he was the person others approached to solve their problems. His cancer diagnosis prompted him to reevaluate his life. Antonio recognized that he was working too many hours and wanted to spend more time with his children and wife. He always had a dream of owning his own restaurant, but never pursued it because he felt like it was too much of a risk to start his own business.

Linda, a 52-year-old Jewish woman of Eastern European ancestry, lives in an affluent suburb of New York City. She was diagnosed 2.5 years ago with stage III breast cancer and endured a double mastectomy and reconstruction, followed by radiation and chemotherapy. When in active treatment, she focused on coping with treatment side effects (i.e., nausea, hair loss, fatigue, body image concerns from the mastectomy) while attempting to maintain a stable family life with her husband, a partner in a prestigious investment banking firm, and her two high-school-aged children. Linda is a pediatrician who joined a small private practice to give her flexibility in balancing work and child rearing. She had a strong support system of friends and neighbors who stepped up to help during her treatment (e.g., bringing in meals, providing transportation to doctors' appointments, and listening to her fears). Linda wanted to protect her children. She felt guilty putting her family through such stress, but she knew rationally that she had no control over that. She could not understand why she got sick. She spent her life taking care of others through her career as a pediatrician, as a loving and caring mother and partner, and an empathic and generous friend. Often she asked, "Why me? I am a good person." Her religious background had emphasized that God punishes the wicked and rewards those who are good. She spent endless hours ruminating about what she had done in her life that led to her illness. The cancer experience caused Linda to reflect on the big questions she always avoided. Her brush with death led her to consider whether she was happy in her life and with her relationships. Over the years she had grown distant from her husband who often worked 7 days a week. He was not emotionally available to her during the illness and she worried that they would become even less intimate because of changes to her body after surgery. She also believed that her kids felt abandoned by her and that her colleagues were frustrated that she had been away from the office so much. At the same time, she was exhausted trying to be a superwoman. Linda realized that she was eating poorly, felt tired much of the time, and was fighting with her husband, in the rare times they were together, because she perceived he was not helping sufficiently.

Aside from skin cancer, breast cancer is the most frequently diagnosed cancer in women and prostate cancer, the most frequently diagnosed in men. Breast cancer treatments, particularly mastectomy and side effects of chemotherapy, can challenge a woman's sense of her femininity (Chang, 2013; Johansen, Andrews, Haukanes, & Lilleaas, 2013) and side effects of prostate cancer treatment (e.g., erectile dysfunction, urinary incontinence, hot flashes) can challenge a man's sense of his masculinity (Grunfeld, Drudge-Coates, Rixon, Eaton, & Cooper, 2013). Both diseases are highly treatable if diagnosed early and both are associated with sexualized body parts, making them useful examples for comparing how males and females come to understand their experiences with cancer. The meaning that patients assign to the various phases of the cancer journey depends on numerous factors such as gender, age, level of education, employment status, and cancer type. Specific findings from the latest research will be discussed. The chapter concludes with applications of existential and relational–cultural therapy (RCT) to the cases of Antonio and Linda.

CANCER AS A TRAUMATIC EXPERIENCE

In many ways cancer represents a prototypical traumatic event; it often strikes without warning, and despite medical advances, the causes are unidentified and the progression is unpredictable (Thornton, 2002). In addition, treatments (e.g., bone marrow transplantation, disfiguring surgeries, chemotherapy, and radiotherapy) are often more debilitating than the disease itself, and have been described by patients as traumatizing (Naidich & Motta, 2000). A cancer diagnosis can be shocking and disruptive. It raises fear of one's mortality and uncertainty about the future, exposes one to invasive procedures and treatments, and causes changes in body image and social relationships (Stanton, Bower, & Low, 2006). Cancer continues to evoke anxiety and dread despite advances in curative and palliative treatments, undermining one's sense of control and challenging assumptions that the world is a safe, fair, and just place. Moser et al. (2014) found that a majority (61%) of Americans, particularly those with low education, continue to perceive cancer as a death sentence, thus adding to the traumatic impact of the diagnosis.

Western medicine has identified over 100 different types of cancer that have unique symptoms, diagnostic procedures, treatments, and mortality rates (National Cancer Institute, 2015). During the course of a lifetime, women in the United States have a one in three chance and men a one in two chance of developing cancer (American Cancer Society, 2016a,b). The estimated number of new cases of invasive cancer expected in the United States in 2016 is 1,655,210 (843,820 women and 841,390 men; American Cancer Society, 2016a,b).

How the illness experience is appraised, experienced, and coped with typically differs across phases (i.e., acute, extended survival, permanent survival). In the acute phase (diagnosis through the first year), adjustment to diagnosis, critical medical decisions, and treatment are the focus. Individuals commonly experience depression and anxiety that tend to dissipate by the end of the year (Andersen & Doyle-Mirzadeh, 1993). Treatment may also severely compromise quality of life during this phase due to invasive surgeries or chemotherapy agents that cause hair loss, fatigue, nausea, and vomiting. Pain, impaired physical and sexual functioning, and low energy are also common (Bloom, 2002). Cognitions are more likely to be intrusive and ruminative in nature during the early stages of trauma, and research has shown that during diagnosis and active treatment, patients with cancer are typically attending to immediate medical issues and juggling life responsibilities (e.g., Park, Edmondson, Fenster, & Blank, 2008). During primary treatment, when participants are dealing with medical decisions and side effects, adaptive coping tends to be problem focused as patients are forced to confront the immediate demands of the situation (e.g., Jim, Richardson, Golden-Kreutz, & Anderson, 2006).

The 3 years following the acute phase is known as the extended survival phase (Bloom, 2002). Impaired functioning and body image changes, greater focus on interpersonal issues, and reestablishment of parental and work roles tend to predominate (Bloom, 2002). As patients move into the posttreatment period, survivors become more reflective (Park et al., 2008; Stanton et al., 2000).

During the subsequent permanent survival phase, the objective probability of recurrence begins to diminish for most cancers. However, fear of recurrence or development of new cancers is common among patients and, for many, may persist indefinitely. Many individuals resume prior activities including employment and recreation despite treatment aftereffects such as loss of energy, cognitive impairment, and relationship issues (Bloom, 2002). Specific meanings derived from the illness experience vary over these phases and may not be clear until long after treatment has ended (e.g., Moadel et al., 1999; Tomich & Helgeson, 2002).

Although cancer diagnoses and treatment are undeniably distressing, research that focuses solely on negative effects provides a limited and potentially inaccurate portrait. Although many individuals with cancer report significant distress during and soon after the diagnostic period (Zabora, BrintzenhofeSzoc, Curbow, Hooker, & Piantadosi, 2001), the majority of survivors eventually return to previous levels of adjustment (Hoskins, 1997) and ultimately report positive change and growth (e.g., Bellizzi & Blank, 2006; Harding, Sanipour, & Moss, 2014). Growth or positive change has been characterized as a greater appreciation for life, more authentic and satisfying interpersonal relationships, a more optimistic view of new possibilities, and a greater spiritual awareness (e.g., Lelorain, Bonnaud-Antignac, & Florin, 2010). Psychological growth has been referred to as stress-related growth, positive psychological change, perceived benefits, and adversarial growth. Although these terms are often used interchangeably and they clearly overlap, research indicates that they may measure different constructs (Stanton & Sears, 2003). For the purposes of this chapter, the growth outcomes after cancer will be conceptualized as posttraumatic growth (PTG).

PTG is thought to occur when a major stressor, such as cancer, is sufficiently unsettling that it challenges one's assumptions about oneself and the world (Tedeschi & Calhoun, 1996) and leads to "cognitive restructuring, search for meaning, and rebuilding of a more positive life perspective" (Arpawong, Richeimer, Weinstein, Elghamrawy, & Milam, 2013, p. 397). PTG can be viewed as a type of a transformative learning experience. Transformative learning is typically instigated by disequilibrium created by an existential crisis (Krouse & Krouse, 1981) or a disorienting dilemma (Mezirow, 2000) that results in a richer and more authentic life. Deriving meaning from reinterpreting the cancer experience is thought to facilitate PTG (e.g., Bellizzi & Blank, 2006), but it can also lead to maladaptive rumination if negative meanings are constructed (Harper et al., 2007).

Meaning Making: Survivors of Cancer

Park et al. (2008) investigated the role of meaning making in psychological adjustment of cancer survivors in the context of coping with life stress. Two distinct components of the meaning-making process were delineated: meaning-making efforts and meanings made (e.g., Gillies & Neimeyer, 2006). This framework defines meaning making as involving efforts to understand a stressor (appraised meaning) and to integrate that understanding into one's global meaning system to reduce the discrepancy between meaning making of cancer and meaning making in general (Park & Folkman, 1997). Park et al. (2008) found that meaning-making efforts were related to better psychological adjustment through the successful creation of adaptive meanings. The meaning making inherent in adaptive thinking helped to reduce rumination and increase psychological well-being.

Most research on meaning making and PTG has been conducted with samples of women with breast cancer, thus making the comparison between genders difficult. Bellizzi and Blank (2006) investigated different facets of PTG and their relationship to demographic and disease and treatment-related factors. In a sample of 224 breast cancer survivors, the researchers found that demographic factors (i.e., marital and employment status, education level, perceived intensity of the disease, and age), as well as coping style, accounted for significant variance in PTG. PTG was reflected in improved interpersonal relationships, openness to new possibilities, and greater appreciation for life. Optimism and hope were not related to PTG. Women with lower education reported higher levels of PTG, but this finding warrants further empirical investigation. Women with invasive breast cancer reported more growth in interpersonal relationships and purpose in life than women with localized cancer. Interestingly, severity of disease did not impact appreciation for life, leading the authors to speculate that beneficial changes on this domain may only require receiving a cancer diagnosis, regardless of the severity.

Research strongly supports positive psychological change in cancer survivors (e.g., Bellizzi & Blank, 2006; Zemore, Rinholm, Shepel, & Richards, 1989). Among women with breast cancer specifically, Stanton et al. (2006) found deep reflection often led to a greater appreciation of life and closer alignment of identity with personal, educational, and career goals. Breast cancer survivors also reported greater spirituality, religious satisfaction, and optimism (Andrykowski et al., 1996; Cordova, Cunningham, Carlson, & Andrykowski, 2001), and more prioritization of themselves and their needs (Thibodeau & MacRae, 1997) as a result of their experience with cancer. As noted by Thornton (2002), cancer survivors report increased independence, inner strength, and enhanced self-worth (e.g., Dirksen, 1995), as well as perceived skills, resources, and attributes (e.g., Calhoun & Tedeschi, 2006).

Breast cancer survivors also reported closer and more authentic interpersonal relationships and the discarding of relationships that were not supportive (Stanton et al., 2006). Andrykowski, Brady, and Hunt (1993) noted that half of cancer survivors in their sample reported enhanced relationships with significant others, children, and friends and attributed this increased closeness to their illness. In another study of patients with breast cancer, 64% indicated that their diagnosis had resulted in more loving, close family relationships (Zemore et al., 1989). Patients with cancer also report being surprised that individuals with whom they might not have had a previous close connection may go above and beyond to be available and helpful (Tedeschi & Calhoun, 2004) and that closer friends and family members have failed to offer the degree of support they would have expected. Although some relationships come to an end, others become stronger with the possibility of gaining greater appreciation and satisfaction within these supportive relationships (Cordova, 2008).

Not all research indicates that growth or positive changes occur after facing significant stressors. Frazier and Kaler (2006) conducted three studies to assess whether posttraumatic growth actually occurs following a major stressor. In one of these studies, they found little evidence for the validity of self-reports of growth. Individuals with breast cancer did not report greater life satisfaction, better relationships, more concern for others, or more positive self-images, despite that these are commonly reported positive life changes among survivors of breast cancer and other stressful or traumatic events. The one exception to this trend was that breast cancer survivors did score higher on measures of the importance of spirituality and prayer (see also Andrykowski et al., 1996).

In addition, the cognitive appraisal of a cancer diagnosis as a challenge or a threat closely mirrors the different paths available to cancer survivors. That is, some survivors may opt to concentrate on the residual effects of the disease and treatment, along with the daily worry regarding the threat of recurrence. On the other hand, individuals view their survival as opportunities to renew or revise their priorities and pursue different paths in terms of activities, interests, and passions. Threat appraisal was found to be a more significant determinant of PTG than objective measures of cancer severity (e.g., Cordova et al., 2001). This finding is consistent with other studies that have failed to find a significant association with PTG and objective medical factors such as cancer therapies including chemotherapy, radiation, tamoxifen/raloxifene (e.g., Cordova et al., 2001; Tomich & Helgeson, 2004), and type of surgery (e.g., Tomich & Helgeson, 2004). One's subjective interpretation of one's illness and treatment is a much more powerful predictor of psychosocial status than are objective factors.

Research on PTG with cancer diagnoses other than breast cancer is limited. A notable exception is a study by Morris and Shakespeare-Finch (2011) who investigated the impact of cancer type on PTG in survivors of breast, prostate, hematological, and colorectal cancer. They found that breast and prostate cancer survivors reported the highest levels of PTG. Those diagnosed with colorectal and hematological cancer reported significantly lower PTG than those with breast cancer. Researchers also found that those who perceived their diagnosis as more traumatic and reported higher levels of distress also reported higher levels of PTG.

GENDER DIFFERENCES IN POSTTRAUMATIC STRESS DISORDER AND POSTTRAUMATIC GROWTH

Research supports that rates of posttraumatic stress disorder (PTSD) and PTG differ by gender (Vishnevsky, Cann, Calhoun, Tedeschi, & Demakis, 2010). Much of this research relies on self-report data, and women are more likely to report distress than men (Brody, 1999). This raises questions as to whether men are experiencing equivalent levels of distress but are less forthcoming. However, we can only report the research that is available, which indicates modest differences.

A meta-analysis revealed that women had higher rates of PTSD and that the difference in PTSD rates has to do with the specific ways in which men and women cognitively appraise traumatic events (Olff, Langeland, Draijer, & Gersons, 2007; Tolin & Foa, 2006). It has been argued that one's cognitive appraisal is equally or more important than the objective facts of the trauma in terms of predicting one's response (Olff et al., 2007). An appraisal can be summarized as a subjective perception, interpretation, and evaluation of an event (Olff et al., 2007) and is an integral component of deriving meaning from one's experience. Differences in appraisal of loss, threat, harm, or control explain why one person may develop PTSD, whereas another, exposed to the same trauma, may not. In comparison with men, women are reportedly more likely to appraise events as stressful and experience increased distress in reaction to a perceived loss of control (Olff et al., 2007). In addition, women are more likely to report avoidance, intrusive thoughts, horror, and panic.

Although evidence is mixed, women also have reported higher rates of PTG than men (Vishnevsky et al., 2010). A PTG meta-analysis revealed a small to moderate difference in PTG as related to gender, with women tending to experience higher rates of growth when faced with adversity (Vishnevsky et al., 2010). Possible explanations of the higher rates of PTG among women compared with men include (1) an increased tendency for women to ruminate on both positive and negative thoughts (Janoff-Bulman, 2006; Tedeschi & Calhoun, 2004), (2) a greater engagement with social support (Swickert & Hittner, 2009), and (3) a smaller discrepancy between their traditional gender role and their role as patient (Seale & Charteris-Black, 2008). Individuals benefit from receiving support and feedback from sympathetic others after sharing a traumatic experience. Women are more likely to seek out these interpersonal interactions and consequently feel closer to others, gain a new perspective, and feel more capable of coping with their illness. Men, in contrast, tend to view illness as a battle with a potential for success or failure, with failure representing a poised threat to masculinity.

GENDER DIFFERENCES: REACTIONS TO CANCER DIAGNOSIS AND TREATMENT

Masculinity is traditionally associated with stoicism and appearing strong when confronted with an illness; however, men's response to cancer is affected by prior roles, sex-role attitudes, and role models such as family and friends with cancer or in remission (Oliffe, 2006). The degree to which perceptions of masculinity are affected by cancer depends, in part, on how much the illness and its treatments influence everyday functioning (Wall & Kristjanson, 2005). Stereotypical masculine traits of assertiveness, dominance, control, physical strength, and emotional restraint are challenged by the cancer experience. In general, men suffer greater social consequences for engaging in unmasculine or feminine behaviors than women do for engaging in masculine behaviors (Messner, 1988). A qualitative study by Grunfeld et al. (2013) revealed that following treatment for prostate cancer, a number of their participants hid physical impairments, presented a strong self-image, limited discussion of their illness, and expressed anxiety around issues of urinary incontinence.

Although the patient role does not necessarily conflict with a feminine gender role, undergoing breast cancer treatment poses significant challenges to a woman's sense of her own femininity. Losing one's breast(s) to mastectomy, losing one's hair to chemotherapy, and losing one's energy and daily routine to treatment and recovery can initially shatter a woman's self-esteem. Breasts are glorified as a symbol of femininity in the United States (Johansen et al., 2013) and women with breast cancer have reported fears of being less attractive to current or future partners (Kashani, Vaziri, Akbari, Far, & Far, 2014).

Several significant differences have been found with regard to how men and women react to a cancer diagnosis, to treatment, and after treatment. In a large representative sample of over 10,000 patients with cancer, Linden,

Vodermaier, MacKenzie, and Greig (2012) found that women reported higher rates of anxiety and depression than men at diagnosis. These researchers also found that the prevalence of anxiety and depression among women with certain types of cancer was two to three times higher than that seen for men. Most studies on gender differences in pain, fatigue, and depression among patients with various cancers revealed no gender-associated differences in fatigue and depression. Those that did find a difference between genders, reported more fatigue and depression in women (Miaskowski, 2004).

In contrast to the results of the Miaskowski (2004) review, Ernst, Beierlein, Romer, Möller, and Bergelt (2013) found that, overall, women expressed higher anxiety and men higher depression. These authors elaborated on the factors that were associated with distress. In women, factors such as younger age (<50 years) and presence of metastases were associated with increased anxiety. Further, women with breast cancer felt less distressed than women suffering from other types of cancer. In men, both anxiety and depression were related to employment concerns. Men who were employed felt less distressed, pointing to work as an important source of purpose and self-esteem, consistent with gender role expectations.

Also in alignment with traditional gender roles, male patients with cancer reported more emotional stability than their female counterparts (Bhattacharjee, 2014). This may be attributable to men's reluctance to report emotional reactions. Female patients with cancer, especially those with breast cancer, have reported body image concerns, leading to emotional distress, withdrawal from social activities, and perceived loss of attractiveness and sexual desirability. Similarly, a study by Boquiren, Esplen, Wong, Toner, and Warner (2013) found that breast cancer survivors who endorsed greater internalization of traditional gender roles and attitudes and engaged in greater self-surveillance and body shame, reported higher body image disturbance levels and poorer quality of life after treatment.

Although few studies investigated meaning making and cancer, the studies that do exist support no gender differences with respect to patients' desire for help in processing existential factors. For example, Moadel and colleagues' (1999) ethnically diverse, urban sample of 248 male and female patients with cancer did not differ with respect to wanting help with overcoming fears (51%), finding hope (42%), meaning in life (40%), and spiritual resources (39%). They also did not differ with regard to wanting someone to talk to about finding peace of mind (43%), meaning of life (28%), and dying and death (25%). Time since diagnosis ranged from 1 month to

22 years, with approximately half of the participants in active treatment. It is important to note that cancer stage, time since diagnosis, and time since treatment completion vary widely across investigations, which makes it difficult to compare how men and women create meaning during their cancer journeys.

Marital status and presence of children are factors in how individuals cope with cancer. Goldzweig et al. (2009) found that married patients cope better with cancer than unmarried patients, and that married men reported significantly higher levels of spouse support and lower levels of peer support than married women. Ernst et al. (2013) found that fathers of underaged children had greater anxiety than men without underaged children. This may be linked to their role as household breadwinners and anxiety about their responsibility to provide for their families. Women with children did not report increased symptoms of anxiety or depression compared with women without children.

RELATIONAL-CULTURAL THERAPY AND EXISTENTIAL THERAPY FOR TREATING INDIVIDUALS WITH CANCER

Two approaches that have particular relevance for individuals who are endeavoring to make sense of their life-altering experiences with cancer are feminist therapy, particularly RCT, and existential therapy. Existential approaches are flexible and emphasize exploration of meaning in the context of a collaborative therapeutic relationship. Integrating RCT into an existential framework by exploring sociocultural identity and the impact of gender socialization can promote client self-understanding and connection with others.

RCT is a form of feminist therapy developed by Judith Jordan and colleagues at the Stone Center that grew out of the work of Jean-Baker Miller (Duffey & Somody, 2011). It is based on several key principles that are shared by all forms of feminist therapy (Frey, 2013) such as a focus on: (1) strength-based change; (2) a collaborative therapy relationship with an ongoing examination of the power differential between client and therapist; (3) the client's sociocultural identity, particularly gender roles; (4) the impact of the therapist's own sociocultural identity on the therapeutic relationship; and (5) client empowerment (e.g., Enns, 2004).

In contrast to other Western therapeutic models that associate independence and autonomy with mental health, RCT posits that an individual gains a healthier and stronger sense of self through growth-fostering relationships with others (Frey, 2013; Jordan, 2001). According to Jordan (1997), the emotional maturity and "felt sense of self" (p. 15) that occurs as a result of these relationships continually evolves throughout the lifespan as the individual moves toward increasing relational complexity and mutuality. Relationships that foster growth are based on mutual empathy and mutual empowerment, and benefit both individuals (Jordan and Dooley, 2000). Empathy, listening, understanding, and support characterize a relationship with a high level of mutuality. Although connectedness through growth-fostering relationships is viewed as the primary pathway to mature functioning, RCT also emphasizes the important role that individual authenticity plays in this process (Duffey & Somody, 2011). Specifically, through representing oneself honestly within a relationship, an individual comes to know his or her own thoughts and feelings more fully and thus develops a stronger sense of self.

RCT also focuses on the ways in which culturally prescribed sex roles negatively impact the development of a complex and "felt sense of self" in both men and women (Frey, 2013; Jordan, 1997, p. 15). In Western culture, men are at risk of being socialized to compete with others, and to value independence and autonomy over relational connectedness (Bergman, 1995). They may also lack healthy coping mechanisms for dealing with negative internal experiences (Cochran, 2006). In contrast, women may fail to represent themselves authentically with others in response to the socio-cultural pressure to be self-sacrificing and maintain relationships at all costs (Miller & Stiver, 1997).

These socialized sex differences may extend to the ways in which men and women cope with the trauma of a cancer diagnosis. One study that investigated RCT concepts in relation to women coping with cancer found that women who prioritized the needs of others demonstrated fewer self-care behaviors (Sormanti, Kayser, & Strainchamps, 1997). Another study found that women who were in a relationship with a highly mutual partner had higher self-care, agency, and quality of life, and lower levels of depression (Kayser, Sormanti, & Strainchamps, 1999). Thus, RCT may be a particularly well-suited form of therapy to apply to both men and women with a cancer diagnosis. RCT could help male patients with cancer bolster and rely on social support systems to foster a stronger sense of interconnectedness and move them toward psychological health. RCT could help female patients with cancer to represent themselves in an authentic way and engage in supportive relationships that are based on mutuality, thus lowering the risk of depression and increasing self-care behaviors.

Existential therapy has roots in existential philosophy and is based on the work of Binswanger, Yalom, Frankl, and others (Vos, Cooper & Craig, 2015). Although there are numerous types of existential therapies, all are phenomenological and person-centered; however, they may differ in terms of the specific concerns that they address and the degree to which they are structured and directive. However, at the heart of all existential therapy models are a number of key philosophical assumptions: (1) humans crave meaning and purpose, (2) humans have freedom that leads to choice and responsibility, (3) it is psychologically healthier to face life's challenges as opposed to denying or avoiding them, (4) subjective experience should be prioritized in therapy, and (5) our experience is fundamentally embedded in our relationships with others (Vos et al., 2015).

Given the focus on finding meaning in the face of life's challenges, existential therapy is well suited for individuals with cancer. Many patients with cancer reflect on existential concerns such as mortality, purpose in the world, the meaning of life, religiosity, and spirituality (Tedeschi & Calhoun, 1995). These reflections can result in increased appreciation of life (Cella & Tross, 1986), a clearer sense of purpose and outlook (Wyatt, Kurtz, & Liken, 1993), a shift in priorities and goals (Collins, Taylor, & Skokan, 1990), and deeper spirituality (Cordova et al., 2001).

A cancer diagnosis heightens one's awareness of death, and as Yalom (1980) noted, individuals often seek psychotherapy to process concerns triggered by confrontations with the givens of existence. In a meta-analysis on the effect of existential therapies on psychological outcomes, Vos et al. (2015) reviewed research that supports the use of this framework with patients with cancer and trauma survivors. The researchers found that existential therapies have similar or larger effects than alternative nonexistential interventions for patients with cancer. This may be because patients with cancer often report having questions about meaning and identity (e.g., Henoch & Danielson, 2009; Lee, 2008; as cited in Vos et al., 2015). In addition, research supports the idea that finding meaning in life is an essential aspect of the way in which individuals cope with stressful life events (Folkman & Moskowitz, 2000; Park, 2010; Park & Folkman, 1997; as cited in Vos et al., 2015).

CASE APPLICATIONS

Antonio

Antonio was hesitant to speak about personal problems outside the family, but when one of his doctors, who was Latino and understood the cultural taboos, reassured Antonio that he was confronted with an enormously difficult situation and needed support, he made an appointment with an existential therapist who integrated RCT. During one of their first meetings, the therapist explored with Antonio how he felt about their differences (i.e., the therapist was a younger, white female, with higher socioeconomic status and greater privilege). Antonio appreciated this discussion and also that his therapist wanted to understand how his race and ethnicity, age, religious and spiritual beliefs, and gender-role expectations influenced his perspectives on himself and the world.

The therapist's history of her father's cancer experience was reactivated through her work with Antonio. She had to monitor her impulse to push Antonio to eat well, exercise, employ relaxation techniques, and get a second medical opinion, as she knew Antonio might resent forceful suggestions or feel guilty if he did not follow her advice. She sought peer supervision to help her work through her own issues related to illness, survival, and death that were triggered by her work with Antonio so she could be fully present with him.

The therapist invited Antonio to engage in a gender and broader cultural analysis. Antonio concluded that he and his wife fell into traditional cultural and gender roles (she focused on family and home life, he on wage earning), and they had a strong and affectionate marriage supported by deep spirituality. The sexual intimacy they enjoyed before Antonio's surgery diminished and he and his wife eventually sought counseling as a couple where they learned to communicate more openly, draw from their faith, and reconnect with one another. Antonio also learned to draw on his extended family for emotional support and practical assistance with daily activities. This provided needed relief for his wife.

Antonio's experience with cancer provided the opportunity to evaluate his life. Was he living authentically? Were his values reflected in his lifestyle? He was working more than 70 h per week and his work took him away from his wife and children. Antonio wanted to work less and be more present with his nuclear and extended family. He had always dreamed of having his own business. Through discussions with his therapist, Antonio approached his boss about investing in a food truck where he could make his own hours and honor his mother by using her family recipes. This new direction would allow him to spend more time with his children who had volunteered to help him on the truck and be more personally meaningful. Although Antonio still feared a recurrence, he felt more prepared to cope should the cancer return.

Linda

When Linda started therapy after treatment she was grieving the many losses she had suffered. For many weeks she wept in therapy and poured out her feelings about adjusting to her new body, the devastating side effects of chemotherapy and radiation, experiences with friends that disappointed her, her worries about her future health, her distant and conflicted relationship with her husband, and her concerns about how her children were faring. Her therapist listened patiently to her stories and empathized. She knew how critical it was to be deeply engaged with Linda in the here-and-now and encouraged expression of the feelings that Linda had held in to protect her loved ones. She encouraged Linda to speak in the first person, elaborate and provide examples for each topic, and confront her fears. Learning how to tolerate ambiguity and uncertainty was a focus of the therapy.

The strong client–therapist relationship helped Linda to cope with her troubles. Linda knew that her therapist would be there for her as she took risks to explore her identity, express her anxieties, search for new meaning and direction, and put into action what she discovered. Linda's illness forced her to think about who she is and what she wants and created an urgency to find meaning and live more authentically. The therapist did not tell Linda what her meaning should be, but pointed out how meaning is often created through suffering. As Linda felt helpless and powerless, the therapist helped her realize that small steps (even simply coming to the office for sessions) demonstrated her ability to choose how to respond to this traumatic experience.

Linda's therapist helped her to explore how her gender-role socialization was affecting her coping strategies. She learned that she could not always sacrifice for others and that she had to pay more attention to her own self-care which meant making time for yoga, eating right, doing mindfulness training, and sleeping more. She considered the cancer a wake-up call and an opportunity to make life-affirming changes. Always a spiritual person, the cancer made her more so. She initiated conversations with her rabbi to discuss her interpretation that illness was a punishment from God. The rabbi referred her to the book, *When Bad Things Happen to Good People,* which provided comfort and helped her to reconnect with her religion. Once Linda viewed God as benevolent she saw cancer as less of a threat and more of an opportunity to grow. The temple community had provided substantial tangible and emotional support through her treatment period and Linda was appreciative. She less frequently sweated the small stuff and tried to keep the focus on caring for herself and her children. Through discussions with the therapist, Linda realized that she was staying with her husband for the sake of the children and because she did not think she had the energy to separate their socially and financially intertwined lives. Linda found the motivation to try a trial separation from her husband and consider whether she wanted to work on repairing her marriage.

As Linda enjoyed expressing herself through writing, the therapist encouraged her to start a gratitude journal. Each night before bed she wrote about the best part of her day and one thing she was grateful for. This activity made a significant difference in Linda's perspective on herself and the world. Clearly, Linda ultimately was able to articulate how she benefitted from her experience with cancer but she was appreciative that her therapist did not see her as somehow deficient because she could not initially articulate how the illness had instigated personal growth. She had needed a safe place to express and explore her distress and not be rushed to positively reframe her experience. Linda perceived that her therapist was fully present, although the therapist acknowledged in her own supervision that it was difficult at times to sit with Linda in her anxiety and sadness as it triggered the therapist's own anxiety about her health and mortality.

CONCLUSION

Women with cancer have been found to be more likely to appraise events as stressful, experience a perceived loss of control, and report more intrusive thoughts, body image concerns, anxiety, avoidance, and distress, whereas men report more emotional stability and potentially higher rates of depression. Women with cancer, particularly those with breast cancer, also report higher levels of PTG than men with cancer. As research on meaning making among patients with cancer is typically based on self-report data, it is difficult to say whether the gender differences identified in the chapter are based on differences in self-disclosure by men and women or differences in lived experiences with cancer.

According to the gender similarity hypothesis, males and females are actually far more similar than different regarding most psychological topics (Hyde, 2005). Empirical investigations of gender differences and similarities proliferated following Hyde's hypothesis, and although Zell, Krizan, and Teeter's (2015) meta-synthesis using data from over 20,000 individual studies found a relatively small overall difference between males and females across multiple domains in psychological science, the researchers "caution against the conclusion that gender differences are trivial or non-existent" (p. 18). It is possible that the way in which males and females create meaning from their experience with cancer may vary more based on individual factors such as age, education level, and social support than based on gender. These individual differences, including cultural background, must been taken into consideration in the mental health care of patients with cancer.

Lastly, there is a dearth of knowledge about gender differences in meaning making and cognitive appraisal at the diagnosis and treatment stages of cancer. Further research is needed to assess gender differences in patients' understanding of cancer; for example, whether they interpret cancer as a threat versus challenge, resulting in potential harm versus growth and how this impacts coping. This information would assist medical professionals and caregivers to better serve their patients with cancer.

REFERENCES

American Cancer Society. (2016a). *Lifetime risk of developing or dying from cancer*. Retrieved from www.cancer.org.

American Cancer Society. (2016b). *Cancer facts and figures 2016*. Atlanta: American Cancer Society.

Andersen, B. L., & Doyle-Mirzadeh, S. (1993). Breast disorders and breast cancer. In D. E. Steward, & N. L. Stotland (Eds.), *Psychological aspects of women's healthcare* (pp. 425–446). Washington, DC: American Psychiatric Press.

Andrykowski, M. A., Brady, M. J., & Hunt, J. W. (1993). Positive psychosocial adjustment in potential bone marrow transplant recipients: cancer as psychosocial transition. *Psycho-oncology, 2*, 261–276.

Andrykowski, M. A., Curran, S. L., Studts, J. L., Cunningham, L., Carpenter, J. S., McGrath, P. C., … Kenady, D. E. (1996). Psychosocial adjustment and quality of life in women with breast cancer and benign breast problems: a controlled comparison. *Journal of Clinical Epidemiology, 49*, 827–834.

Arpawong, T. E., Richeimer, S. H., Weinstein, F., Elghamrawy, A., & Milam, J. E. (2013). Posttraumatic growth, quality of life, and treatment symptoms among cancer chemotherapy outpatients. *Health Psychology, 32*, 397–408.

Bellizzi, K. M., & Blank, T. O. (2006). Predicting posttraumatic growth in breast cancer survivors. *Health Psychology, 25*, 47–56.

Bergman, S. J. (1995). Men's psychological development: a relational perspective. In R. F. Levant, & W. S. Pollack (Eds.), *A new psychology of men* (pp. 68–90). New York, NY: Basic Books.

Bhattacharjee, A. (2014). Emotional control of cancer patients: a comparative investigation. *Journal of Psychosocial Research, 9*, 19–26.

Bloom, J. R. (2002). Surviving or thriving? *Psycho-Oncology, 11*(2), 89–92.

Boquiren, V. M., Esplen, M. J., Wong, J., Toner, B., & Warner, E. (2013). Exploring the influence of gender-role socialization and objectified body consciousness on body image disturbance in breast cancer survivors. *Psycho-Oncology, 22*, 2177–2185. http://dx.doi.org/10.1002/pon.3271.

Brody, L. (1999). *Gender, emotion, and the family*. Cambridge, Mass: Harvard University Press.

Calhoun, L. G., & Tedeschi, R. G. (2006). The foundations of posttraumatic growth: an expanded framework. In L. G. Calhoun, & R. G. Tedeschi (Eds.), *Handbook of posttraumatic growth: Research and practice* (pp. 3–23). Mahwah, NJ: Erlbaum.

Cella, D. F., & Tross, S. (1986). Psychological adjustment to survival from Hodgkin's disease. *Journal of Consulting and Clinical Psychology, 54*, 616–622.

Chang, F. (2013). Expressive arts and breast cancer: Restoring femininity. In C. A. Malchiodi, & C. A. Malchiodi (Eds.), *Art therapy and health care* (pp. 146–161). New York, NY: Guilford Press.

Cochran, S. V. (2006). Struggling for sadness: a relational approach to healing men's grief. In M. Englar-Carlson, & M. A. Stevens (Eds.), *In the room with men: A casebook of therapeutic change* (pp. 91–107). Washington, DC: American Psychological Association.

Collins, R. L., Taylor, S. E., & Skokan, L. A. (1990). A better world or a shattered vision? Changes in perspectives following victimization. *Social Cognition, 8*, 263–285.

Cordova, M. J. (2008). Facilitating posttraumatic growth following cancer. In P. A. Linley, & S. Joseph (Eds.), *Trauma, recovery, and growth: Positive psychological perspectives on posttraumatic stress*. Hoboken, NJ: Wiley & Sons.

Cordova, M. J., Cunningham, L. L. C., Carlson, C. R., & Andrykowski, M. A. (2001). Posttraumatic growth following breast cancer: a controlled comparison study. *Health Psychology, 20*, 176–185.

Dirksen, S. R. (1995). Search for meaning in long-term cancer survivors. *Journal of Advanced Nursing, 21*, 628–633.

Duffey, T., & Somody, C. (2011). The role of relational-cultural theory in mental health counseling. *Journal of Mental Health Counseling, 33*, 223–242.

Enns, C. Z. (2004). *Feminist theories and feminist psychotherapies: origins, themes, and diversity* (2nd ed). Binghamton, NY: Haworth Press.

Ernst, J. C., Beierlein, V., Romer, G., Möller, B., & Bergelt, C. (2013). Use and need for psychosocial support in cancer patients: a population-based sample of patients with minor children. *Cancer, 119*, 2333–2341.

Folkman, S., & Moskowitz, J. T. (2000). Positive affect and the other side of coping. *American Psychologist, 55*, 647–654.

Frazier, P. A., & Kaler, M. E. (2006). Assessing the validity of self-reported stress-related growth. *Journal of Consulting and Clinical Psychology, 74*, 859–869.

Frey, L. L. (2013). Relational-cultural therapy: theory, research, and application to counseling competencies. *Professional Psychology: Research and Practice, 44*, 177.

Gillies, J., & Neimeyer, R. A. (2006). Loss, grief, and the search for significance: toward a model of meaning reconstruction in bereavement. *Journal of Constructivist Psychology, 19*, 31–65.

Goldzweig, G., Andritsch, E., Hubert, A., Walach, N., Perry, S., Brenner, B., & Baider, L. (2009). How relevant is marital status and gender variables in coping with colorectal cancer? A sample of middle-aged and older cancer survivors. *Psycho-Oncology, 18*, 866–874.

Grunfeld, E. A., Drudge-Coates, L., Rixon, L., Eaton, E., & Cooper, A. (2013). The only way I know how to live is to work: a qualitative study of work following treatment of prostate cancer. *Health Psychology, 32*, 75–82. http://dx.doi.org/10.1037/a0030387.

Harding, S., Sanipour, F., & Moss, T. (2014). Existence of benefit finding and posttraumatic growth in people treated for head and neck cancer: a systematic review. *PeerJ, 2013*(1). http://dx.doi.org/10.7717/peerj.256.

Harper, F. W. K., Schmidt, J. E., Beacham, A. O., Salsman, J. M., Averill, A. A., Graves, K. D., & Andrykowski, M. A. (2007). The role of social cognitive processing theory and optimism in positive psychosocial and physical behavior change after cancer diagnosis and treatment. *Psycho-oncology, 16*, 79–91.

Henoch, I., & Danielson, E. (2009). Existential concerns among patients with cancer and interventions to meet them: an integrative literature review. *Psycho-Oncology, 18*(3), 225–236. http://dx.doi.org/10.1002/pon.1424.

Hoskins, C. N. (1997). Breast cancer treatment-related patterns in side effects, psychological distress, and perceived health status. *Oncology Nursing Forum, 24*, 1575–1583.

Hyde, J. S. (2005). The gender similarities hypothesis. *American Psychologist, 60*, 581–592. http://dx.doi.org/10.1037/0003-066X.60.6.581.

Janoff-Bulman, R. (2006). Schema-change perspectives on posttraumatic growth. In L. G. Calhoun, & R. G. Tedeschi (Eds.), *Handbook of posttraumatic growth: Research and practice* (pp. 81–99). Mahwah, NJ: Erlbaum.

Jim, H. S., Richardson, S. A., Golden-Kreutz, D. M., & Andersen, B. L. (2006). Strategies used in coping with a cancer diagnosis predict meaning in life for survivors. *Health Psychology, 25*(6), 753–761.

Johansen, V. F., Andrews, T. M., Haukanes, H., & Lilleaas, U. (2013). Symbols and meanings in breast cancer awareness campaigns. *NORA: Nordic Journal of Women's Studies, 21*(2), 140–155. http://dx.doi.org/10.1080/08038740.2013.797024.

Jordan, J.V. (1997). A relational perspective for understanding women's development. *Women's growth in diversity: More writings from the Stone Center*, 9–24.

Jordan, J. V. (2001). A relational-cultural model: healing through mutual empathy. *Bulletin of the Menninger Clinic, 65*, 92–103.

Jordan, J. V., & Dooley, C. (2000). *Relational practice in action: A group manual*. Wellesley, MA: Stone Center Publications.

Kashani, F. L., Vaziri, S., Akbari, M. E., Far, Z. J., & Far, N. S. (2014). Sexual skills, sexual satisfaction and body image in women with breast cancer. *Procedia – Social and Behavioral Sciences, 159*, 206–213. http://dx.doi.org/10.1016/j.sbspro.2014.12.358. In *5th World Conference on Psychology, Counseling and Guidance, WCPCG-2014, May 1–3 2014*. Dubrovnik, Croatia.

Kayser, K., Sormanti, M., & Strainchamps, E. (1999). Women coping with cancer: the influence of relationship factors on psychosocial adjustment. *Psychology of Women Quarterly, 23*, 725–739.

Krouse, H. J., & Krouse, J. H. (1981). Cancer as crisis: the critical elements of adjustment. *Nursing Research, 31*, 96–101.

Lee, V. (2008). The existential plight of cancer: meaning-making as a concrete approach to the intangible search for meaning. *Supportive Care in Cancer, 16*, 779–785. http://dx.doi.org/10.1007/s00520-007-0396-7.

Lelorain, S., Bonnaud-Antignac, A., & Florin, A. (2010). Long-term posttraumatic growth after breast cancer: prevalence, predictors and relationships with psychological health. *Journal of Clinical Psychology in Medical Settings, 17*, 14–22. http://dx.doi.org/10.1007/s10880-009-9183-6.

Linden, W., Vodermaier, A., MacKenzie, R., & Greig, D. (2012). Anxiety and depression after cancer diagnosis: prevalence rates by cancer type, gender, and age. *Journal of Affective Disorders, 141*, 343–351.

Messner, M. (1998). The limits of the male sex role: an analysis of the men's liberation and men's rights movements' discourse. *Gender & Society, 12*, 255–276.

Mezirow, J. (2000). Learning to think like an adult. In J. Mezirow, & Associates (Eds.), *Learning as transformation: Critical perspectives on a theory in progress* (pp. 3–34). San Francisco, CA: Jossey-Bass.

Miaskowski, C. (2004). Gender differences in pain, fatigue, and depression in patients with cancer. *Journal of the National Cancer Institute Monographs, 32*, 139–143.

Miller, J. B. (1986). *Toward a new psychology of women* (2nd ed.). Boston, MA: Beacon.

Miller, J. B., & Stiver, I. P. (1997). *The healing connection: How women form relationships in therapy and in life*. Boston: Beacon Press.

Moadel, A., Morgan, C., Fatone, A., Grennan, J., Carter, J., Laruffa, G., … Dutcher, J. (1999). Seeking meaning and hope: self-reported spiritual and existential needs among an ethnically-diverse cancer patient population. *Psycho-Oncology, 8*, 378–385.

Morris, B., & Shakespeare-Finch, J. (2011). Cancer diagnostic group differences in posttrau-matic growth: accounting for age, gender, trauma severity, and distress. *Journal of Loss and Trauma, 16*, 229–242.

Moser, R. P., Arndt, J., Han, P. K., Waters, E. A., Amsellem, M., & Hesse, B. W. (2014). Percep-tions of cancer as a death sentence: prevalence and consequences. *Journal of Health Psy-chology, 19*, 1518–1524.

Naidich, J. B., & Motta, R. W. (2000). PTSD-related symptoms in women with breast cancer. *Journal of Psychotherapy in Independent Practice, 1*, 35.

National Cancer Institute. (2015). *Lifetime risk of developing or dying from cancer.* Retrieved from http://www.cancer.gov/about-cancer/understanding/what-is-cancer.

Olff, M., Langeland, W., Draijer, N., & Gersons, B. P. (2007). Gender differences in posttrau-matic stress disorder. *Psychological Bulletin, 133*, 183–204.

Oliffe, J. (2006). Embodied masculinity and androgen deprivation therapy. *Sociology of Health & Illness, 28*, 410–432. http://dx.doi.org/10.1111/j.1467-9566.2006.00499.x.

Park, C. L. (2010). Making sense of the meaning literature: An integrative review of meaning making and its effects on adjustment to stressful life events. *Psychological Bulletin, 136*, 257–301.

Park, C. L., Edmondson, D., Fenster, J. R., & Blank, T. O. (2008). Meaning making and psy-chological adjustment following cancer: the mediating roles of growth, life meaning, and restored just-world beliefs. *Journal of Consulting and Clinical Psychology, 76*, 863–875.

Park, C. L., & Folkman, S. (1997). Meaning in the context of stress and coping. *General Review of Psychology, 1*, 115–144.

Seale, C., & Charteris-Black, J. (2008). The interaction of class and gender in illness narratives. *Sociology, 42*, 453–469.

Sormanti, M., Kayser, K., & Strainchamps, E. (1997). A relational perspective of women cop-ing with cancer: a preliminary study. *Social Work in Health Care, 25*, 89–106.

Stanton, A., Bower, J. E., & Low, C. A. (2006). Posttraumatic growth after cancer. In L. G. Calhoun, & R. G. Tedeschi (Eds.), *Handbook of posttraumatic growth: Research and practice* (pp. 138–175). Mahwah, NJ: Erlbaum.

Stanton, A. L., Danoff-Burg, S., Cameron, C. L., Bishop, M., Collins, C. A., Kirk, S. B., & Tillman, E. (2000). Emotionally expressive coping predicts psychological and physical adjustment to great cancer. *Journal of Counseling and Clinical Psychology, 68*, 875–882.

Stanton, A. L., & Sears, S. (2003). Benefit finding in women with early stage breast cancer. In *Paper presented at the 24th annual society of behavioral medicine conference. Salt lake city, Utah.*

Swickert, R., & Hittner, J. (2009). Social support coping mediates the relationship between gender and posttraumatic growth. *Journal of Health Psychology, 14*, 387–393.

Tedeschi, R. G., & Calhoun, L. G. (1995). *Trauma and transformation: Growing in the aftermath of suffering.* Thousand Oaks, CA: Sage.

Tedeschi, R. G., & Calhoun, L. G. (1996). The posttraumatic growth inventory: measuring the positive legacy of trauma. *Journal of Traumatic Stress, 9*, 455–471.

Tedeschi, R. G., & Calhoun, L. G. (2004). Posttraumatic growth: conceptual foundations and empirical evidence. *Psychological Inquiry, 15*, 1–18.

Thibodeau, J., & MacRae, J. (1997). Breast cancer survival: a phenomenological inquiry. *Advances in Nursing Science, 19*(4), 65–74.

Thornton, A. A. (2002). Perceiving benefits in the cancer experience. *Journal of Clinical Psy-chology in Medical Settings, 9*, 153–165.

Tolin, D. F., & Foa, E. B. (2006). Sex differences in trauma and posttraumatic stress disorder: a quantitative review of 25 years of research. *Psychological Bulletin, 132*, 959–992.

Tomich, P. L., & Helgeson, V. S. (2002). Five years later: a cross-sectional comparison of breast cancer survivors with healthy women. *Psycho-Oncology, 11*(2), 154. http://dx.doi.org/10.1002/pon.570.

Tomich, P. L., & Helgeson, V. S. (2004). Is finding something good in the bad always good? Benefit finding among women with breast cancer. *Health Psychology, 23*, 16–23.

Vishnevsky, T., Cann, A., Calhoun, L. G., Tedeschi, R. G., & Demakis, G. J. (2010). Gender differences in self-reported posttraumatic growth: a meta-analysis. *Psychology of Women Quarterly, 34*, 110–120. http://dx.doi.org/10.1111/j.1471-6402.2009.01546.x.

Vos, J., Craig, M., & Cooper, M. (2015). Existential therapies: a meta-analysis of their effects on psychological outcomes. *Journal of Consulting and Clinical Psychology, 83*(1), 115–128. http://dx.doi.org/10.1037/a0037167.

Wall, D., & Kristjanson, L. (2005). Men, culture and hegemonic masculinity: understanding the experience of prostate cancer. *Nursing Inquiry, 12*, 87–97. http://dx.doi.org/10.1111/j.1440-1800.2005.00258.x.

Wyatt, G., Kurtz, M., & Liken, M. (1993). Breast cancer survivors: an exploration of quality of life issues. *Cancer Nursing, 16*(6), 440–448.

Yalom, I. D. (1980). *Existential psychotherapy.* New York: Basic Books.

Zabora, J., BrintzenhofeSzoc, K., Curbow, B., Hooker, C., & Piantadosi, S. (2001). The prevalence of psychological distress by cancer site. *Psycho-Oncology, 10*, 19–28.

Zell, E., Krizan, Z., & Teeter, S. R. (2015). Evaluating gender similarities and differences using metasynthesis. *American Psychologist, 70*, 10–20. http://dx.doi.org/10.1037/a0038208.

Zemore, R., Rinholm, J., Shepel, I., & Richards, M. (1989). Some social and emotional consequences of breast cancer and mastectomy: a content analysis of 87 interviews. *Journal of Psychosocial Oncology, 7*(4), 33–45.

CHAPTER 5

Forgiveness Therapy in the Reconstruction of Meaning Following Interpersonal Trauma

N. Wade[1], J.M. Schultz[2], M. Schenkenfelder[1]
[1]Iowa State University, Ames, IA, United States; [2]Augustana College, Rock Island, IL, United States

At the time of his initial interview, Mike[1] was a 35-year-old Hispanic male working as a university professor. His paternal great-grandparents and maternal grandparents both emigrated from Mexico. Mike identified as Mexican-American and was proud of both his Mexican and American cultural heritage. He was raised and is currently residing in the upper Midwest region of the United States. Mike reported that he had significant problems through his adolescent and young adult life, consisting of risky sexual behaviors, explosive anger, and depression, as well as dissociation, emotional dysregulation, and suicide attempts consistent with borderline personality disorder.

Growing up, Mike experienced significant abuse, mostly from his father. Mike reported early memories (as young as 4 or 5 years old) of feeling despised by his father. Most of the traumatic experiences were physically violent and emotionally abusive. For example, Mike described how his father would drag him by his hair and throw him against walls when he was angry. Common punishments for misbehavior included being whipped on bare skin with branches or belts; on several occasions he remembers bleeding from these whippings. Despite these brutal physical traumas, Mike recalled that the emotional abuse felt equally traumatic. He recalled the ways his father would belittle him in front of his siblings and friends, how he would mock both his efforts to do well (e.g., laughing at a picture drawn by Mike) and his experience of pain (e.g., being laughed at and mimicked when crying). He also reported significant experiences of being yelled and screamed at for reasons he could not understand or predict. In addition to creating psychological distress, this abuse had a considerable impact on his

---

[1] The client's name, demographic information, and some treatment details have been changed to protect identity.

Reconstructing Meaning After Trauma
ISBN 978-0-12-803015-8
http://dx.doi.org/10.1016/B978-0-12-803015-8.00005-X

69

developing meaning system. His view of the world and himself was obviously shaped by these negative experiences, and as a child he experienced very limited hope for the future and purpose for his life.

Growing up, Mike had a history of religious participation as a Catholic. In his early 20s he moved away from organized religion. However, in his late 20s, Mike began exploring meditation and through that developed a personal Buddhist practice and life outlook. One of the basic tenets of Buddhism is compassion for others and the cultivation of loving-kindness. As Mike developed these more he realized the potential benefit of being able to bring these to his childhood abuse and worked toward developing compassion for his family, in particular his father. Ultimately, he was able to achieve a degree of forgiveness for his family that went beyond just tolerating the memories of the hurt and offenses, so that his forgiveness deepened his recovery and growth and opened broader access to meaning in his life.

However, Mike did not come to forgive his family through religion alone. Psychological treatment, including traditional trauma work and specific forgiveness intervention, was instrumental in his recovery and development at various points in his life. His initial work in therapy did not specifically address forgiveness; instead, he worked with a therapist to come to terms with the horrible ways he had been mistreated and to alleviate the host of symptoms he experienced as a result. Later in his recovery, explicitly addressing forgiveness in a therapy group led by the first author allowed him to explore forgiveness as a therapeutic goal. That forgiveness work then became a considerable part of his ability to recreate the meaning that had been so severely arrested in his childhood.

It is well known that traumatic experiences, including interpersonal traumas like Mike experienced, can dramatically alter people's understanding of the world and negatively affect their sense of meaning (Janoff-Bulman, 2002). Recovery from these difficult experiences includes rebuilding broken assumptions about the self and the world. One way that people might be able to rebuild their lives and seek meaning following interpersonal trauma is through forgiveness. In this chapter, we examine forgiveness as a potential mechanism for meaning making with a focus on clinical implications.

FORGIVENESS

As the research on forgiveness has grown, definitions have been offered, critiqued, and refined. Although no complete consensus exists, researchers working with people who have experienced traumatic interpersonal offenses are working toward a shared understanding of forgiveness. At a basic level, these researchers seem to agree that forgiveness is an intrapersonal process that includes reduction in anger and bitterness and some increase in or return to a positive state toward the offending person (e.g., Freedman & Enright, 1996; Greenberg, Warwar, & Malcolm, 2008; Harris et al., 2006; Wade, Worthington, & Haake, 2009). Many have made the point that forgiveness is not the same as reconciliation; people can forgive others without returning to a trusting relationship with them (e.g., because the person is not trustworthy, has moved away, or has died; Worthington, 2006). In addition, forgiveness is different from condoning the hurtful actions of another person, forgetting the hurt, or minimizing the negative effects of the offense (Enright, 2001).

Instead, forgiveness includes an acknowledgement of the pain and suffering caused and may allow for justice to be served. Despite being forgiven, significant offenses might never be forgotten. Thus, for the purposes of this chapter, we define forgiveness as a process that occurs internal to the person who was offended against in which they experience less anger, hurt, bitterness, and/or vengefulness, and a return to preoffense levels of benevolence, compassion, and/or love. Furthermore, this forgiveness occurs without giving up important interpersonal boundaries that can keep the offended person safe from future harm (Wade, Bailey, & Shaffer, 2005).

For Mike, forgiveness meant letting go of the anger he had toward his father and moving toward more benevolent feelings. Eventually, he was able to develop empathy for his father, to acknowledge how his father's own childhood abuse had contributed to his abusive behavior. This empathy allowed for some compassion and hope that his father might seek out help of his own. However, forgiveness did not mean that Mike would forget the trauma caused by his father or view his father's actions as acceptable or somehow justified. Forgiveness also meant that Mike did not let his own children be alone with his father; he did this out of a genuine desire to protect his children and not to spite his father or to express anger or bitterness.

MEANING MAKING

Park's (2010) model of meaning making suggests that people possess global meaning systems that help us understand our experiences and the world. Global meaning comprises (1) beliefs about the self and world (e.g., predictability, controllability, benevolence of humanity), (2) goals (e.g., companionship, self-acceptance, financial security, achievement), and (3) a general sense of meaning or purpose. When faced with a stressor or trauma, individuals make appraisals related to the situational meaning of the event (e.g., why did it happen, degree of threat and controllability). Individuals experience distress when global meaning and situational appraisals are discrepant; this distress then initiates a process of meaning making.

The meaning-making process may entail a variety of strategies to resolve the discrepancy between global meaning and situational appraisals (Park, 2010). Forgiveness can either help people engage these strategies or be seen as a meaning-making strategy in its own right. As such, forgiveness might serve as a mechanism of meaning making, an important part of the journey from trauma to meaning for many people.

FORGIVENESS AND MEANING MAKING

The Forgiveness Process Model, a prominent and well-supported theoretical model of forgiveness, illustrates how forgiveness and meaning making are connected (Enright & Fitzgibbons, 2000). Within the model, forgiveness is theorized to encompass four phases: uncovering, decision, work, and deepening. During the deepening phase, individuals find meaning from their experience and may develop a new purpose, mirroring outcomes of the meaning-making process (Park, 2010). In the Forgiveness Process Model, meaning making is a key component of forgiveness; we suggest that forgiveness may also be important in facilitating meaning making for some.

As a coping tactic specific to interpersonal offenses and traumas, some have conceptualized forgiveness as a meaning-making strategy (Finnegan, 2010; Grossman, Sorsoli, & Kia-Keating, 2006). Folkman (1997) identified positive reappraisal, modification of goals and planning goal-directed problem-focused coping, and mobilizing spiritual beliefs as general strategies for meaning making. Within this (1997) framework, forgiveness may serve as a problem-focused coping strategy to improve distress and/or relationships. For some, forgiveness may also be situated within a spiritual or religious framework. Both of these were certainly true in Mike's case. Mike was only able to access the possibility of forgiveness through his spiritual worldview informed by Buddhism. Without his beliefs about compassion and the oneness of all being, he would have had much less motivation to even consider forgiveness. Once he had the motivation, forgiveness became an additional way for him to cope with the fallout from his traumatic experiences.

Specifically, he came to see forgiveness as a gift that he could give to himself, to his father and family, and ultimately to the universe. By viewing forgiveness as his gift, he was better able to cope with his trauma and the symptoms resulting from it, feeling a strong sense of meaning in his forgiveness work.

Forgiveness may directly facilitate achievement of meaning making in a variety of ways. Common outcomes of the meaning-making process include renewed sense of meaning or purpose in life, understanding the cause of the event (reattribution), altered global beliefs, changed global goals, and post-traumatic growth (Park, 2010). With regard to the first outcome, research suggests that forgiveness predicts an increased sense of meaning in life over time, and continually offering forgiveness buffers the deleterious impact on meaning when individuals experience multiple offenses (Van Tongeren et al., 2015).

Second, through the process of seeking to better understand and develop empathy for the offender, an individual may reattribute the cause of the event thereby reducing discrepancy between global meaning and situational appraisal. In Mike's case, forgiveness helped him to rework appraisals that the traumatic offenses happened because he was a worthless son and that his father was an evil, despicable man. He was able to develop more compassion and empathy for his father by considering his father's own abusive childhood without excusing his father's horrific behaviors. In this way, the empathy-building component of forgiveness can be seen as a crucial step toward the broader outcome of meaning development.

Third, changing global meanings to reduce the discrepancy caused by the stressor (accommodation) is another way to reduce the discrepancy between global meaning and situational appraisal (Joseph & Linley, 2005). Victims of interpersonal traumas may have many global beliefs challenged by their experiences. The process of forgiveness, while focused on the specific event and relationship, may help individuals shift the global meanings to more closely align with their experiences, particularly through the development of empathy and compassion.

Fourth, although much of the research has focused on violation of global beliefs, goals are also an important component within the meaning-making model. In fact, the violation of goals through the experience of a trauma may be the more significant meaning-making predictor of psychological adjustment (Park, Mills, & Edmondson, 2012; Steger, Owens, & Park, 2015). Relational goals, including strivings for affiliation and intimacy, have been identified as among the most common across individuals (Emmons, 1999, 2003). Although forgiveness is an intrapersonal process, it may facilitate these interpersonal goals, particularly following an interpersonal trauma. If an interpersonal trauma shattered the global goal of being close with one's family, forgiveness may facilitate reconciliation. For individuals who pursue forgiveness but not reconciliation with the perpetrator, releasing anger and bitterness through forgiveness may provide for deeper support and connection in other relationships.

Again, these insights are illustrated in Mike's experience. Mike struggled with relationships as a result of his trauma. He felt a painful tension between getting too close to others (fearing he would lose himself) and being too far away (fearing that he might lose those important to him). This led Mike to engage in many counterproductive behaviors, such as dismissing the needs of people close to him and demanding to know where significant others were at all times. Through forgiveness he was able to see his own relational needs and goals in a new context and to understand that others might be able to meet those needs without abusing him. Although intimate relationships were still painful and difficult at times for him, forgiveness allowed him more freedom to work toward his goal of being close to others.

FORGIVENESS AND POSTTRAUMATIC GROWTH

Posttraumatic growth, which may be the most common benefit of meaning making (Park et al., 2012), is defined as finding benefit or experiencing growth as a result of a struggle with a stressful or challenging experience (Tedeschi & Calhoun, 1995, 2004). Areas of posttraumatic growth include changes in perception of self, improved interpersonal relationships, altered life philosophy, changes in religion and spirituality, and new directions in life (Affleck & Tennen, 1996; Linley & Joseph, 2004; Tedeschi & Calhoun, 1995, 2004). Cognitive processing is believed to play a key role in the achievement of posttraumatic growth through restructuring beliefs and assumptions challenged by the stressor (Tedeschi & Calhoun, 1995, 2004).

Conceptually, there is significant overlap in the constructs of posttraumatic growth and forgiveness. Although forgiveness is sometimes identified as an emotion-focused coping strategy (Worthington & Scherer, 2004; Worthington & Wade, 1999), forgiveness therapy encourages the individual to also engage in significant cognitive processing of the event (e.g., remembering the impact, seeking to understand motives of the offender), which may also spawn posttraumatic growth. Achieving forgiveness also has the potential to facilitate posttraumatic growth, particularly in the domains of improved interpersonal relationships and changes in religion and spirituality for individuals who situate forgiveness in a religious or spiritual framework.

Empirical support for the relationship between forgiveness and post-traumatic growth to date is largely supportive. Research suggests that forgiveness predicts posttraumatic growth in individuals who have experienced a range of significant interpersonal offenses (Heintzelman, Murdock, Krycak, & Seay, 2014; Schultz, Tallman, & Altmaier, 2010; Wusik, Smith, Jones, & Hughes, 2015). Experimental evidence shows that writing about the benefits of an interpersonal offense or benefits of forgiveness (i.e., identifying posttraumatic growth) causes increases in forgiveness (Crowley, 2014; McCullough, Root, & Cohen, 2006). In support of the conceptual relationship described earlier, cognitive processing played an important role in the effects of the benefit-finding conditions on forgiveness in both these studies. However, some studies have found no relationship (Fischer, 2006) or unclear qualitative relationships between the constructs (McCormack & Sly, 2013; Nguyen et al., 2014).

Religion and spirituality may play an important and complex role in the relationship between posttraumatic growth and forgiveness. The personal importance of religion has been shown to mediate the relationship between forgiveness and posttraumatic growth (Schultz et al., 2010) and forgiveness interventions have facilitated posttraumatic growth in religion and spirituality (Luskin, Ginzburg, & Thoresen, 2005; Rye & Pargament, 2002). However, in a nonintervention study, forgiveness did not predict spiritual growth in adults (Schultz, Altmaier, Ali, & Tallman, 2014).

After his 20s, Mike began to see the damage his anger and bitterness was doing to his life. He connected this insight to his growing awareness of Buddhist teachings through his practice of meditation. Mike reported that when he turned 30 he reached a decision to work on himself, which included exploring his past experiences and the impact these had on him. Then after 2 years of individual therapy and much progress toward reducing his explosive anger, suicidal tendencies, and learning ways to regulate strong emotion, Mike heard about a forgiveness treatment group that was being offered. Mike joined the group and made considerable progress. Thus, in Mike's case, the abuse spawned posttraumatic spiritual growth in developing connection to his Buddhist practice, which then provided a strong basis for his pursuit of forgiveness.

INTERVENTIONS TO PROMOTE FORGIVENESS

If forgiveness after an interpersonal trauma facilitates posttraumatic growth and meaning making, then we should be motivated to effectively promote forgiveness, and in turn the meaning-making process, in clinical settings. Clinically oriented researchers started testing interventions to help people forgive past hurts in the early 1990s (e.g., DiBlasio & Benda, 1991; Hebl & Enright, 1993). The prevailing conclusion from these studies is that forgiveness interventions are effective for helping people to develop forgiveness and reduce depression and anxiety (Wade, Hoyt, Kidwell, & Worthington, 2014). In their meta-analysis of 53 forgiveness intervention studies (2323 total participants), Wade and colleagues found an overall effect size of 0.56 when interventions were compared with no treatment. When compared with an alternative treatment, the effect size was 0.45, favoring the forgiveness treatments. Furthermore, they found evidence consistent with a dose–response relationship found by Worthington et al. (2000), who reported that the duration of explicit forgiveness interventions correlated strongly with treatment effect size (0.70–0.86 depending on the studies included).

Although there is some variation in what occurs in forgiveness interventions, a common core to these interventions has been described (Wade & Worthington, 2005). In general, most interventions to promote forgiveness include several broad elements: (1) helping clients talk about the offense(s) in a safe, emotionally contained environment; (2) providing opportunities for clients to gain empathy for the offending person; (3) helping clients to understand and make a commitment to forgiveness; and (4) offering ways to cope with and reduce anger, bitterness, and other aspects of unforgiveness.

Research in this area is limited in several ways. No research has yet been done to understand when the topic of forgiveness should be addressed in therapy. In one study, more psychotherapy sessions predicted the desire to talk about forgiveness with one's individual therapist (Wade et al., 2005). Although this might suggest that clients tend to be more comfortable approaching the topic of forgiveness later in therapy, we do not yet know if waiting longer in therapy to approach the topic of forgiveness is beneficial to clients.

Another important issue that is not fully addressed in the research on forgiveness interventions is understanding when a client is seeking true forgiveness or a pseudoforgiveness that comes from self-blame that often involves excusing or minimizing the offense, and may result in the victim of trauma remaining in abusive situations without establishing healthy boundaries. Obviously, these are not desirable outcomes for people who have experienced interpersonal trauma.

In addition, research on forgiveness therapy does not directly address the issue of whether forgiveness increases meaning following trauma or whether psychological interventions might help people to recover by addressing the meaning-making process. Despite this current limitation in the research, the work reviewed that makes the connection between forgiveness and meaning provides a viable direction for future research on recovery from traumatic interpersonal events.

IMPLICATIONS FOR RESEARCH AND PRACTICE

Research: One of the main questions about the connection between forgiveness and meaning is to what degree forgiveness serves as a mechanism in the development of meaning following trauma. We have tried to suggest ways in which forgiveness might be an important part of the process from traumatic interpersonal experiences to the development of meaning, but empirical research has not established this as a causal link. Relatedly, the temporal unfolding of the forgiveness and meaning-making processes is unclear. Does forgiveness facilitate meaning making or vice versa? Research has also not directly and rigorously tested if forgiveness therapies produce meaning in clients. There may also be important cultural variations in these processes that should be studied and better understood, including, but not limited to, religious and spiritual identity. More work on the role of forgiveness in meaning making would help to answer this question and further direct clinical work in this area. Another important implication of this review is that more applied research could be conducted to help practitioners know more about what makes forgiveness therapy an effective tool for achieving positive outcomes such as meaning making and posttraumatic growth. Specifically, questions of when to offer forgiveness interventions could be answered through surveys and interview studies of clients who have forgiven offenders (and those who have not). Exploration of when those clients felt prepared to tackle forgiveness, how that preparation came about, and what recommendations they have for helping clients in the future could establish a deeper foundation of knowledge in this area. This research would be well complimented by similar research with experienced clinicians, particularly those who are open to forgiveness interventions. Surveying a broad range of therapists would also help, from those doing private practice with higher functioning clients to those in community mental health agencies.

Research addressing questions related to pseudoforgiveness is also needed. Knowledge could be expanded in the area of what predicts the likelihood of someone engaging in pseudoforgiveness and how those factors might be mitigated. Application of existing psychotherapeutic interventions to help reduce pseudoforgiveness would also be worth-while. For example, could Emotion-Focused Therapy (Greenberg, 2002) or Acceptance and Commitment Therapy (Hayes & Smith, 2005) tech-niques be used effectively to help clients recognize and accept their feel-ings of anger, rejection, bitterness, and desires for justice?

Practice: This review also suggests important implications for practice. First, clinicians should consider offering forgiveness work to their clients who have been hurt. Research supports the efficacy and benefit of these interventions (Wade et al., 2014). However, this work should be offered after clients have had opportunities to explore their hurts and access the self-protective emotions of anger and justice. For some clients, forgiveness interventions may need to wait; for others, forgiveness may be the primary need. To assess for readiness, clinicians might focus on the client's emotional, cognitive, and behavioral reactions to the offense. What is the client feeling, thinking, and doing in response to being hurt? Does the client have ways of protecting himself/herself, can the client identify the negative implications of the hurt without overly blaming herself/himself, and does the client avoid condoning or minimizing the offense? If yes, these are good indica-tions that the client may be ready for forgiveness intervention.

Another important implication for practice is identifying pseudofor-giveness and making efforts to short-circuit this process. Helping clients to see that they may be missing out on important information by ignoring or downplaying their self-protective emotions can be an important step toward true forgiveness. This includes helping clients to see that to truly forgive another person there must be some real offense to be forgiven. If the hurt was minimal, justified for some reason, or caused by the client, then there really is nothing to forgive. Instead, forgiveness grows out of an awareness of injustice and acceptance of anger and any bitterness, vengefulness, or hatred that may have resulted from the hurt. Once these have been explored, accepted, and felt, then the client can make steps toward forgiving the offending person, when they are ready to do so.

Finally, helping clients to see the meaning in their forgiveness can be especially helpful for the healing process. Clients who can connect the act of forgiving to some higher purpose will likely have both an easier time working on forgiveness and more additional positive outcomes to forgiving. There are several different meanings that clients might attach to their for-giveness. Some clients may see forgiveness primarily as a way to heal and to protect themselves from being victim to the negative effects of long-term bitterness. Their health and well-being is more important than their anger and bitterness, so they have the will to forgive to help themselves. Other clients might hold personal or religious values that encourage forgiveness. Therefore, they are motivated to work toward forgiveness because they see this as a higher calling in their life.

Whatever the meaning is, it may be important for clinicians to help clients explore the purpose of their forgiveness. Likewise, clients may also find it valuable to see how forgiving can increase the meaning they have in their lives. Forgiveness may be a part of the process that helps them repair the damage to their worldview and view of self that the trauma caused. As Mike said following his own work on forgiveness, "Now that I can forgive my father, I see that I have options for even the worst things people can do to me. Life can be cruel at times, but I have choices. Forgiveness is now one of those choices."

CONCLUSION

Through the forgiveness work that Mike accomplished, he was able to create a new aspect to meaning in his life. Although he had developed some sources of meaning as a young adult (e.g., being athletic, charity work), none of those old sources of meaning related to his childhood. Now, he had developed both a worldview (i.e., compassion for all) and a source of meaning making in his life (i.e., forgiving those who hurt him) that was relevant to his entire life. His forgiveness went beyond just the specific traumatic events of his past and developed into a model for the way he wanted to live his life. He had found a powerful way to cope with wrongs done to him: true forgiveness that allowed him to release anger and still hold the offending person accountable, develop strong boundaries against future hurts, show compassion even for the most hurtful people, and restore meaning.

REFERENCES

Affleck, G., & Tennen, H. (1996). Construing benefits from adversity: adaptational significance and dispositional underpinnings. *Journal of Personality, 64*, 899–922.

Crowley, J. P. (2014). Expressive writing to cope with hate speech: assessing psychobiological stress recovery and forgiveness promotion for lesbian, gay, bisexual, or queer victims of hate speech. *Human Communication Research, 40*, 238–261.

DiBlasio, F. A., & Benda, B. B. (1991). Practitioners, religion and the use of forgiveness in the clinical setting. *Journal of Psychology and Christianity, 10*(2), 166–172.

Emmons, R. A. (1999). *The psychology of ultimate concerns: Motivation and spirituality in personality.* New York: The Guilford Press.

Emmons, R. A. (2003). Personal goals, life meaning, and virtue: wellsprings of a positive life. In C. Keyes, & J. Haidt (Eds.), *Flourishing: Positive psychology and the life well-lived* (pp. 105–128). Washington, DC: American Psychological Association.

Enright, R. D. (2001). *Forgiveness is a choice: A step-by-step process for resolving anger and restoring hope.* Washington, D.C: American Psychological Association.

Enright, R. D., & Fitzgibbons, R. P. (2000). *Helping clients forgive: An empirical guide for resolving anger and restoring hope.* Washington, DC: American Psychological Association.

Finnegan, A. C. (2010). Forging forgiveness: collective efforts amidst war in northern Uganda. *Sociological Inquiry, 80,* 424–447.

Fischer, P. C. (2006). *The link between posttraumatic growth and forgiveness: An intuitive truth. Handbook of posttraumatic growth: Research & practice.* Mahwah, NJ: Lawrence Erlbaum Associates Publishers, 311–333.

Folkman, S. (1997). Positive psychological states and coping with severe stress. *Social Science & Medicine, 45,* 1207–1221.

Freedman, S. R., & Enright, R. D. (1996). Forgiveness as an intervention goal with incest survivors. *Journal of Consulting and Clinical Psychology, 64,* 983–992.

Greenberg, L. S. (2002). *Emotion-focused therapy: Coaching clients to work through feelings.* Washington, DC: American Psychological Association.

Greenberg, L. S., Warwar, S. H., & Malcolm, W. M. (2008). Differential effects of emotion-focused therapy and psychoeducation in facilitating forgiveness and letting go of emotional injuries. *Journal of Counseling Psychology, 55,* 185–196.

Grossman, F. K., Sorsoli, L., & Kia-Keating, M. (2006). A gale force wind: meaning making by male survivors of childhood sexual abuse. *American Journal of Orthopsychiatry, 76,* 434–443.

Harris, A., Luskin, F., Norman, S. B., Standard, S., Bruning, J., Evans, S., & Thoresen, C. E. (2006). Effects of a group forgiveness interventions on forgiveness, perceived stress, and trait-anger. *Journal of Clinical Psychology, 62,* 715–733.

Hayes, S. C., & Smith, S. (2005). *Get out of your mind and into your life: The new acceptance and commitment therapy.* Oakland, CA: New Harbinger.

Hebl, J., & Enright, R. D. (1993). Forgiveness as a psychotherapeutic goal with elderly females. *Psychotherapy: Theory, Research, Practice, Training, 30*(4), 658–667.

Heintzelman, A., Murdock, N. L., Krycak, R. C., & Seay, L. (2014). Recovery from infidelity: differentiation of self, trauma, forgiveness, and posttraumatic growth among couples in continuing relationships. *Couple and Family Psychology: Research and Practice, 3,* 13–29.

Janoff-Bulman, R. (2002). *Shattered assumptions: Towards a new psychology of trauma.* New York: The Free Press: New York.

Joseph, S., & Linley, P. A. (2005). Positive adjustment to threatening events: an organismic valuing theory of growth through adversity. *Review of General Psychology, 9*(3), 262–280.

Linley, P. A., & Joseph, S. (2004). Positive change following trauma and adversity: a review. *Journal of Traumatic Stress, 17,* 11–21.

Luskin, F. M., Ginzburg, K., & Thoresen, C. E. (2005). The efficacy of forgiveness intervention in college age adults: randomized controlled study. *Humboldt Journal of Social Relations, 29,* 163–184.

McCormack, L., & Sly, R. (2013). Distress and growth: the subjective "lived" experience of being the child of a Vietnam veteran. *Traumatology, 19,* 303–312.

McCullough, M. E., Root, L. M., & Cohen, A. D. (2006). Writing about the benefits of an interpersonal transgression facilitates forgiveness. *Journal of Consulting and Clinical Psychology, 74,* 887–897.

Nguyen, C. M., Liu, W. M., Phan, T. T., Pittsinger, R., Casper, D., & Alt, R. (2014). Vietnamese military men's perceptions of the long-term psychological effects of reeducation camps. *Psychology of Men & Masculinity, 15,* 407–418.

Park, C. L. (2010). Making sense of the meaning literature: an integrative review of meaning making and its effects on adjustment to stressful life events. *Psychological Bulletin, 136,* 257–301.

Park, C. L., Mills, M. A., & Edmondson, D. (2012a). PTSD as meaning violation: testing a cognitive worldview perspective. *Psychological Trauma: Theory, Research, Practice, and Policy, 4,* 66–73.

Park, C. L., Riley, K. E., & Snyder, L. B. (2012b). Meaning making coping, making sense, and post-traumatic growth following the 9/11 terrorist attacks. *Journal of Positive Psychology, 7,* 198–207.

Rye, M. S., & Pargament, K. I. (2002). Forgiveness and romantic relationships in college: can it heal the wounded heart? *Journal of Clinical Psychology, 58,* 419–441.

Schultz, J. M., Altmaier, E., Ali, S., & Tallman, B. (2014). A study of posttraumatic spiritual transformation and forgiveness among victims of significant interpersonal offences. *Mental Health, Religion & Culture, 17,* 122–135.

Schultz, J. M., Tallman, B. A., & Altmaier, E. M. (2010). Pathways to posttraumatic growth: the contributions of forgiveness and importance of religion and spirituality. *Psychology of Religion and Spirituality, 2,* 104–114.

Steger, M. F., Owens, G. P., & Park, C. L. (2015). Violations of war: testing the meaning-making model among Vietnam veterans. *Journal of Clinical Psychology, 71*(1), 105–116.

Tedeschi, R. G., & Calhoun, L. G. (1995). *Trauma and transformation: Growing in the aftermath of suffering.* Thousand Oaks, CA: Sage.

Tedeschi, R. G., & Calhoun, L. G. (2004). Posttraumatic growth: conceptual foundations and empirical evidence. *Psychological Inquiry, 15,* 1–18.

Van Tongeren, D. R., Green, J. D., Hook, J. N., Davis, D. E., Davis, J. L., & Ramos, M. (2015). Forgiveness increases meaning in life. *Social Psychological and Personality Science, 6,* 47–55.

Wade, N. G., Bailey, D., & Shaffer, P. (2005). Helping clients heal: does forgiveness make a difference? *Professional Psychology: Research and Practice, 36,* 634–641.

Wade, N. G., Hoyt, W. T., Kidwell, J. E. M., & Worthington, E. L., Jr. (2014). Efficacy of psychotherapeutic interventions to promote forgiveness: a meta-analysis. *Journal of Consulting and Clinical Psychology, 82*(1), 154–170.

Wade, N. G., & Worthington, E. L., Jr. (2005). In search of a common core: a content analysis of interventions to promote forgiveness. *Psychotherapy: Theory, Research, Practice, Training, 42,* 160–177.

Wade, N. G., Worthington, E. L., Jr., & Haake, S. (2009). Promoting forgiveness: comparison of explicit forgiveness interventions with an alternative treatment. *Journal of Counseling and Development, 87,* 143–151.

Worthington, E. L., Jr. (2006). *Forgiveness and reconciliation: Theory and application.* New York: Brunner-Routledge.

Worthington, E. L., Jr., Kurusu, T. A., Collins, W., Berry, J. W., Ripley, J. S., & Baier, S. N. (2000). Forgiving usually takes time: a lesson learned by studying interventions to promote forgiveness. *Journal of Psychology and Theology, 28,* 3–20.

Worthington, E. L., Jr., & Scherer, M. (2004). Forgiveness is an emotion-focused coping strategy that can reduce health risks and promote health resilience: theory, review, and hypotheses. *Psychology & Health, 19,* 385–405.

Worthington, E. L., & Wade, N. G. (1999). The social psychology of unforgiveness and forgiveness and implications for clinical practice. *Journal of Social and Clinical Psychology, 18,* 385–418.

Wusik, M. F., Smith, A. J., Jones, R. T., & Hughes, M. (2015). Dynamics among posttraumatic stress symptoms, forgiveness for the perpetrator, and posttraumatic growth following collective trauma. *Journal of Community Psychology, 43,* 389–394.

CHAPTER 6

Spiritually Oriented Psychotherapy for Trauma and Meaning Making Among Ethnically Diverse Individuals in the United States

G.E.K. Allen, P.S. Richards, T. Lea
Brigham Young University, Provo, UT, United States

Esmeralda, a 42-year-old Latina woman from Mexico, had moved to the United States with hopes of a bright new future. Despite not knowing much English, she had worked hard, found and married her husband, and had several beautiful children. She missed her family in Mexico, but loved living in the United States. At least, she had liked it up until the day her 5-year-old son was hit and killed by a truck only a few feet from where she stood. The accident had changed everything. In an instant, Esmeralda went from being a caring and involved mother to barely being able to be physically or emotionally present with her children. Two years after her son's death, Esmeralda presented for treatment with Dr. T. In her first session, she acknowledged that she was struggling with debilitating depression and that it had left her unable to get out of bed for days at a time.

Esmeralda's entire family had witnessed her son's death and they were all suffering. For example, Esmeralda was perplexed about how to handle her 10-year-old son's behavioral problems at school. She was troubled by her husband's lack of interest in their marriage. She was experiencing fear and guilt about her teenage daughter's suicide threats. She explained how ashamed and hopeless she felt when her daughter's teacher said, "If you don't get it together you are going to lose another one of your children to suicide."

It was after her conversation with the teacher that Esmeralda reached out to her religious community. Esmeralda was raised Roman Catholic and the Catholic Church in her area welcomed her and her family. Their family

Reconstructing Meaning After Trauma
ISBN 978-0-12-803015-8
http://dx.doi.org/10.1016/B978-0-12-803015-8.00006-1
83

began attending church regularly and Esmeralda attended a weekend retreat with some other women from her church. It was at the retreat that Esmeralda began healing. She told Dr. T that while on the retreat she felt God's love for her and reassurance that He had a plan for her and her family. She explained it was this spiritual experience that gave her the hope to pursue treatment.

After Esmeralda opened up to Dr. T about her son's accident, Dr. T spent several sessions with helping her work through the grief and rage she felt about his traumatic death. Partway through this working through process, Esmeralda began one of her therapy sessions by asking Dr. T if she could tell him about a dream she had experienced the previous week.

Esmeralda related that during her dream she found herself in a shining white kitchen. She had never seen the kitchen before, but knew it was her kitchen. After entering her kitchen, she started making tortillas. As she worked, she heard her young deceased son enter the room, sit on the floor, and begin playing with his small cars. As he played and she worked, she explained that a sense of normalcy and peace entered her heart. She glanced at her son every so often, but nothing felt out of place or strange. She explained that it was like he had always been with her. She said the peace she was feeling seemed to last for several hours.

Then, suddenly, Esmeralda said that three tall angels came into the kitchen and told her son it was time to go. The young boy stood up and started to leave the kitchen. As she saw him leaving, Esmeralda said it felt as if the entire 2 years of grief she had experienced since his death came crashing down on her. Terror ripped through her body and she screamed at him to stay. She said that her son stopped, turned around, and approached her. He explained that he was going to be okay, and without another word, turned and left the room.

Dr. T asked Esmeralda what she made of her dream. She said she believed it was her son's spirit that had come to say good-bye. She explained how thoughtful her son had been in life, even at a small age. She said she knew he had come to give her one last sweet memory together, a memory they could both cherish. She said she could finally put to rest her worry that he was still suffering. She found solace in her belief that he was in heaven.

Dr. T told Esmeralda that he felt it would be important for her to hold on to this memory. He recommended that Esmeralda write the dream down and share it with her family, if she felt it was appropriate to do so. Dr. T recommended that she reach out to her religious community and talk more with her Bishop about her experience. Dr. T also recommended that

Esmeralda pray for help to hold onto the feelings she had experienced during the dream.

The dream was a turning point in Esmeralda's treatment. It assuaged the traumatic pain she had been feeling. She reported for the first time in 2 years being able to see her family's dire situation with clarity. She started being more physically and emotionally present with her children. Over time, Dr. T treated her 10-year-old son and teenage daughter, and had one large family session with all of her children and her husband. After Esmeralda's dream, her family's progress was remarkable.

Esmeralda's dream and personal spirituality—and the support she and her family received from their Bishop and religious community—were powerful resources during treatment and recovery. Dr. T felt privileged to be a witness to the healing power of faith and spirituality in his work with Esmeralda and her family.

In this chapter, the effectiveness of spiritually oriented psychotherapy for trauma and meaning making among religious ethnically diverse individuals is explored. We begin the chapter with a case example to illustrate the role spirituality can play in treatment and recovery from trauma. We briefly discuss relevant research findings that provide evidence of the relationship between trauma and spirituality. We mention several process guidelines for implementing spiritual treatment approaches. We then discuss the application of spiritual approaches with racial ethnic minority groups in the United States and cultural influences to meaning making and healing. We conclude by offering several recommendations for research and training in this domain.

EMPIRICAL CONNECTIONS BETWEEN TRAUMA AND SPIRITUALITY

There is growing empirical evidence that trauma of all kinds can have a devastating impact on individual's religious faith and sense of spiritual well-being. Like the case of Esmeralda, traumatic events reach into a person's life, unbidden, and shatter the basic assumptions that life is safe, that people can be trusted, and that justice exists (Grant, 1999; Herman, 1997). For those individuals who are religiously minded the basic assumptions of safety, trust, and justice were often built into their core religious beliefs. The trauma survivor was taught these assumptions as a child or believed them as an adult; therefore, trauma not only challenges a survivor's basic assumptions of how the world works, but can also challenge his or her fundamental religious beliefs. Ryan's (1998) in-depth qualitative study of 50 women who had experienced sexual, emotional, and/or physical violence before age 19 years concurred with this notion in that she found that almost half of the women had no current religious affiliation. Seventy-five percent of the women had been raised in a religious home, but had left the religion of their childhood to either pursue a different religion or other forms of spirituality.

For those that suffer a decrease in their religious affiliation due to the shattering effects of trauma, an increased susceptibility to psychological distress is often found. In a survey of 608 individuals who had lost a friend or loved one in the September 11, 2001, terrorist attacks on the twin towers, Seirmarco et al. (2012) found that the 11% of respondents that self-reported a decrease in their religious beliefs were almost three times more likely to screen positive for complex grief, two and a half times more likely to have major depressive disorder, and two times more likely to have posttraumatic stress disorder.

Religious affiliations are not the only component of spirituality that can be affected by experiencing a traumatic event. Weber and Cummings (2003) survey of 158 upper-level university students showed that those students who had experienced physical, sexual, or emotional abuse as a child showed a lower level of existential well-being, which is described as having a clear sense of personal meaning and direction in life. Pritt's (1998) comparative study of 115 women belonging to the Church of Jesus Christ of Latter-day Saints, who were sexually abused as children, and 70 women who had not reported any such abuse, provides further evidence that one's spirituality can suffer after a traumatic event. In this study the group of women that had been sexually abused as children reported that core assumptions about self, others, and the world had been damaged by the abuse, the abuse had also created a feeling of alienation from self and from God, and their ability to find personal meaning in life had been severely damaged.

As illustrated in the case example of Esmeralda, there is also growing evidence that religious faith and spiritual practices can help trauma survivors cope, heal, and recover. Often the most important coping skill for trauma survivors is finding meaning in the traumatic experience (Frankl, 2006; Grant, 1999; Herman, 1992). Even though an individual's spirituality is often damaged by a traumatic event, many trauma survivors view their recovery as a spiritual journey (Blakley, 2007). In the qualitative study of 50 women, mentioned earlier, who had experienced sexual, emotional, and/or physical violence before age 19 years, they found that even though half had no religious orientation and 75% had left the religion of their childhood, more than half the women felt their spirituality was stronger because of the spiritual journey they experienced as they came to terms with the violence inflicted on them as children (Ryan, 1998).

Grossman, Sorsoli, and Kia-Keating (2006) also showed in an in-depth qualitative study of 16 male survivors of childhood sexual abuse that the survivors employed three main strategies to make meaning of the violence they had experienced. The survivors made meaning in actions, through thought, and by developing or calling on a sense of spirituality. This type of spiritual coping has been found to be a good predictor of posttraumatic growth. In a survey of 101 survivors of childhood sexual abuse, spiritual coping was the best predictor of lower levels of current trauma symptomology when controlling for demographics, severity of abuse, cognitive appraisal, and support satisfaction (Gall, 2006). It was also found in a qualitative study of 103 rape survivors that ethnicity, positive religious coping, and the interaction between the two were the best predictors of posttraumatic growth after the assault (Ahrens, Abeling, Ahmad, & Hinman, 2010).

In a qualitative survey of 24 inpatients with eating disorder who had experienced various forms of trauma (i.e., sexual abuse, physical abuse, emotional abuse, serious illness, divorce of parents, death of family members), Berrett, Hardman, O'Grady, and Richards (2007) found that patients perceived that the trauma they had experienced had injured their sense of spirituality. Many of the patients also perceived that recovering their faith and sense of spirituality was an important part of their journey toward recovery. This research points to the fact that when dealing with trauma, spirituality can be either the deepest scars or the epicenter of resilience, healing, and recovery.

EMPIRICAL FINDINGS ABOUT SPIRITUALLY ORIENTED PSYCHOTHERAPIES

The number of spiritually oriented psychotherapies described in the mainstream psychological literature has increased dramatically during the past two decades. These approaches encourage clinicians to use interventions that respect the healing potential of their clients' faith traditions and lead to psychological improvement (Richards & Bergin, 2005; Sperry & Shafranske, 2005). This was the situation for Esmeralda in which she was able to return to her religious and spiritual practices and use them in psychotherapy to make meaning in her life and begin her healing process. Spiritual psychotherapies grounded in the theologies of both Western (theistic) and Eastern spiritual traditions have been described in the psychological literature, including Buddhist, Hindu, Christian, Jewish, Muslim, and ecumenical theistic approaches (e.g., Richards & Bergin, 2004, 2005). Spiritual treatment approaches have been used with various multicultural and special client populations, including African Americans, Asian Americans, Latinos(as), Native Americans, gays, lesbians, and bisexuals (Richards & Bergin, 2004, 2014).

Spiritual psychotherapies have been used most frequently in a treatment-tailoring manner during individual psychotherapy with adult clients; however, they have also been used in group therapy, couple and family therapy, and child and adolescent therapy (Richards & Bergin, 2005). Spiritual approaches and interventions have also been applied with many clinical issues, including trauma, and disorders that may have their roots in traumatic experiences, such as depression, anxiety, addictions, eating disorders, and dissociative disorders. Several outcome reviews published during the past two decades have concluded that there is general support for the effectiveness of spiritually oriented treatment approaches (Richards & Worthington, 2010).

GENERAL PROCESS GUIDELINES FOR USING SPIRITUALLY ORIENTED PSYCHOTHERAPY

When Dr. T invited Esmeralda to explore the meaning of her dream with her deceased son, Dr. T was being open to diverse spiritual worldviews so that a safe place of spiritual understanding and meaning could be present for Esmeralda. When using spiritual treatment approaches, therapists should adopt a therapeutic stance that is open to diverse spiritual perspectives and make efforts to learn more about the spiritual beliefs and cultures of their clients. Therapists can establish a spiritually safe and open therapeutic relationship with their clients by letting them know it is permissible and appropriate to explore spiritual issues if they wish. Permission can be given in the written informed consent document given clients at the beginning of treatment, as well as verbally in the initial session, or at other times, if needed. Therapists can let clients know that spirituality is a potential resource in treatment. Asking questions about clients' religious and spiritual backgrounds on an intake questionnaire can also help validate the importance of spirituality and open the door to spiritual discussions. It is important for therapists to communicate interest and respect when clients self-disclose information about their religious tradition and spiritual beliefs.

We recommend that therapists conduct a multidimensional assessment of their clients that includes a religious–spiritual assessment (Richards &

Bergin, 2005). The goal of spiritual assessment is to help therapists and patients understand the patients' spiritual framework so that they can generate an effective treatment plan that is sensitive to the patient's belief system (Richards & Bergin, 2005). When conducting a spiritual assessment, it is helpful to give clients the opportunity to explore and articulate what spirituality means to them. Religious activities and practices such as attending church, reading scriptures, praying, and so on, are potentially important and helpful, but spirituality may mean more. It may also include experiences such as feeling compassion, loving others, accepting love, feeling hope, receiving inspiration, being honest, feeling gratitude, and experiencing a sense of life meaning and purpose. A spiritual assessment with trauma survivors should also include exploring the history of the trauma, how it may have impacted the client's religious faith and personal spirituality, and how the client's spirituality could be a resource in treatment and healing.

Spiritual resources and interventions that are in harmony with clients' beliefs should be used when it appears that this could help clients cope, heal, and change. A variety of spiritual interventions can be used in a culturally sensitive, treatment-tailoring manner. To the extent possible, therapists should tailor their interventions to fit the unique spiritual and cultural beliefs and practices of their clients (Richards & Bergin, 2014). We will say more about this later. Additional information about the connections between trauma, spirituality, and psychotherapy healing can be found in the book *Spiritually Oriented Psychotherapy for Trauma* (Walker, Courtois, & Aten, 2015).

SPIRITUALLY ORIENTED APPROACHES FOR TRAUMA WITH RELIGIOUS ETHNIC MINORITIES IN THE UNITED STATES

Throughout this section, we will discuss spiritually oriented psychotherapies for trauma with ethnic minorities in the United States. Some scholars have focused their research on specific spiritual coping strategies in psychotherapy with persons of color (Allen & Heppner, 2011; Allen & Smith, 2015; Comas-Diaz, 2006). In the past, the literature on psychological and spiritual interventions related to trauma among racial, ethnic minority individuals has focused primarily on Latinos/as, Asian Americans, African Americans, and Native American Indians—groups also represented in general psychology research, which we will address later in this section. However, there is another unique racial, ethnic minority group in the United States that has not been adequately researched and warrants further examination—Polynesians. In this brief part of the chapter, it is necessary that we spend some time addressing basic background information, cultural constructs, and spiritual characteristics of Polynesians to better inform society of this historically underrepresented racial, ethnic group in the United States.

Polynesian Americans have been conspicuously underrepresented in all aspects of psychological and spiritually oriented psychotherapy research. A few studies have examined Native Hawaiians and/or Pacific Islanders in general (McCubbin, 2006; McCubbin, Ishikawa, & McCubbin, 2008), but very little empirical investigation has specifically focused on Polynesian Americans, particularly on their spiritual and psychological well-being in the mainland United States (Allen, Garriott, Reyes, & Hsieh, 2013; Allen & Heppner, 2011). Most of the Polynesians in the United States reside in the western region namely, Hawaii, California, Washington, and Utah (Allen et al., 2013).

For decades Polynesian Americans have been lumped under the broad Asian American/Pacific Islander census category, although they represent a group that is distinct culturally, historically, linguistically, and religiously. Research focused on Polynesian Americans not only provides necessary descriptions of unique cultural characteristics, but also facilitates understanding of specific psychological and spiritual processes in the Polynesian American cultural context (e.g., McCubbin, 2006). Such research is essential to informing culture-specific and spiritually oriented adaptations to psychotherapy (Bernal & Sáez-Santiago, 2006), which have been shown to improve client outcomes in treatment (Griner & Smith, 2006).

In addition, the origins of this people are important in understanding their psychological and spiritual functioning and health. Specifically, Polynesian Americans emigrated from what is known as the Polynesian triangle (Allen et al., 2013; Allen & Heppner, 2011). The triangle, which stretches from New Zealand to Easter Island and then north to Hawai'i, is a concentrated area in the northern, central, and southern areas of the Pacific Ocean that consists of many islands, including Hawai'i, Kingdom of Tonga, Samoa (Western and American), Tahiti, Cook Islands, New Zealand, Fiji, French Polynesia, Easter Island, Marquesas Islands, and others. The word *Polynesian* comes from the Greek word *Polynesia* (*polus*–many and *nesos*–islands), which is the preferred form of identification by those who come from these island groups. Each Polynesian has a unique collectivistic and spiritual culture, which adds to the richness of their collectivistic worldview and their ability to overcome hardships together. Their immigration to the mainland United States and psychological and spiritual processes warrant further investigations.

Only more recently has there been empirical research conducted on the integration of psychotherapy and religiosity/spirituality among Polynesian Americans. Based on empirical investigations for psychotherapy, collectivistic coping for Polynesians in the United States was found to be helpful with trauma and distress involving death or illness of a loved one, breakup of a significant other, and unemployment or job loss. The two most helpful collectivistic coping strategies among Polynesian Americans were receiving emotional support from family and spiritual support from God, church, and congregational/social support, which were also linked to self-acceptance and purpose in life (Allen & Heppner, 2011) as well as pleasant living at home and openness to discussing important matters at home (Allen & Smith, 2015). Similar to Esmeralda's case of spiritually oriented living and behaviors, Polynesians too engage in spiritual practices that buffer trauma, namely, private and communal prayer, fasting, attending holy temples, reading scriptural text, and receiving guidance from ecclesiastical leaders (Allen & Heppner, 2011; Allen & Smith, 2015). Although some research has been documented, further research is needed and warranted for this unique racial, ethnic minority group in the United States around spiritually oriented strategies in psychotherapy for trauma and meaning making.

Another racial, ethnic group that utilizes spiritual and cultural coping strategies in psychotherapy for trauma in the United States is Latinos/as. For many Latinos/as (as in the case of Esmeralda), spiritual healing permeates the Latino life through everyday language with supplications such as, "Si Dios quiere" calling upon God, angels, and spiritual guidance during their daily activities. These cultural-embedded practices instill hope, sustenance, and a purpose to life (Comas-Diaz, 2006). In addition, prayer appears to be not only a spiritually oriented approach to psychotherapy, but also a culturally sensitive and adaptive one for many Latinos. Prayers requesting guidance from earlier saints (common Catholic practice) can be a source of remedy in times of trauma. The concept of *fatalismo* for many Latinos, which is the belief that life's misfortunes are inevitable (i.e., sudden/unexpected deaths), may create a resigned feeling toward fate. However, with prayer and other spiritually oriented and meaning-making strategies, Latinos can more effectively navigate through these fateful feelings and may more effectively and assertively address traumatic challenges (Sue & Sue, 2012). Comas-Diaz (2006) lists several culturally sensitive and spiritually oriented strategies for psychotherapists when working with Latinos and issues of trauma. Some of these are listed below:

- Use of imagery and fantasy in therapy. Cultural heroes and heroines can be utilized for victims of trauma to reimagine protection and safety.
- Religious rituals to destroy the traumatized life and nurture an experience of a new meaningful life such as engaging in communal rosaries, novenas, posadas, peregrinations, and purification ceremonies.

- Honor ancestors by calling on them for wisdom and counsel. It is not uncommon to maintain relationships with loved ones beyond death through dreams, visions, and visitations for additional spiritual assistance.
- Seeking a "Curandera" (traditional Native healer) to receive additional healing for mind and body.

Another practice that may be common among many Latinos/as is *limpia*, a ritual and spiritual cleansing. The curandera conducts this ancient practice by cleansing the client's spirit of illness and suffering. This can be done through a bath with scented herbs and flowers. The client is also encouraged to eat only fruits and vegetables before the limpia. During the limpia, the curandera performs a ritual sweeping over the body with herbs and specific relevant phrases. Ultimately, the ceremony ends with a prayer and the client is given a bundle of herbs as a sign of hope to be made well (Parks, Zea, & Mason, 2014).

Another racial, ethnic minority group that may use spiritually oriented strategies to buffer the effects of trauma is African Americans. For many African American families, religious and spiritual beliefs play an important role in their lives and can facilitate healing from trauma and remedy life's stressors through spiritual coping strategies (Richardson & June, 1997; Sue & Sue, 1999, 2012). Besides clinics, schools, hospitals, or other mental health professionals, another effective source of psychological help from trauma for black Americans is their churches through counseling and support from their pastors, ministers, and congregational members. Furthermore, church provides not only relief from trauma, but also economic support, opportunities for self-expression, leadership, and community involvement, which all can be interconnected to alleviating the affects of trauma (Sue & Sue, 1999, 2012). For example, some qualitative research shows that African American individuals who suffer with trauma due to serious illnesses, including human immunodeficiency virus infection/acquired immune deficiency syndrome, were able to utilize religious/spiritual meaning-making strategies to help them cope with these serious conditions (Jacobson, Luckhaupt, Delaney & Tsevat, 2006). Much of the meaning-making strategies were instilled both at a very early age and currently while in Sunday school, church youth programs, feeling accepted by caring church friends, and thoughts and feelings of appreciation for God (Jacobson et al., 2006). Below are some narrative meaning-making strategies expressed by some African Americans (Jacobson et al., 2006):

I go unto the holy of holies, that mean[s] I forget all about myself, and, I begin to concentrate on God, and I take my mind there, and I, I can visualize Him, and you know, I see him as this light, and that's something I do, I get in his presence. And I can tell a difference, because I feel anointed, I can feel his presence. (p. 45)

It's actually the recovery process that's made me think a lot about God's personality, my relationship with God. I always knew about the Father, Son, and Holy Ghost, but, to be actually introduced to the Spirit, this is like, a new process for me. (p. 48)

I know that they (good things) wouldn't have happened if it wasn't for God. It's like He's put me through a test, and I'm passing it, I'm trying to get my life together, to go to church to show Him my appreciation. (p. 49)

It's not God I don't trust, it's people that I've had such a hard time, all my life, that I don't trust. I don't hate people, I don't like a lot of people's ways, I can't change that, but I love God dearly. (p. 51)

Specifically among African American Christian churches, there are core religious beliefs that help people overcome trauma. Some of these are: God is forgiving and will not burden a person with more than they can bear. He is in charge and has a specific plan for each of us. God is all powerful, fair, and just (Cook & Wiley, 2014; Holt, Lewellyn, & Rathweg, 2005). Psychotherapists who strive to serve this community should incorporate culturally specific interventions (which include spiritually oriented strategies) and become aware and sensitive to the spiritual strength and connection African Americans receive from their belief in God. In addition, external resources such as church activity, support from ecclesiastical leaders, and social and emotional support from congregation members can offer additional assistance during psychotherapy sessions.

For other racial, ethnic minorities, such as Asian Americans, the concept of body and mind are inseparable and both are essential for holistic health. Somatic symptoms expressed through psychological and emotional stress are common and culturally appropriate in psychotherapy (Conrad & Pacquiao, 2005; Sue & Sue, 2012). In addition to this integration of body and mind among Asian Americans, a third piece to the self is spiritual for many in the United States. Although the research around spiritually oriented psychotherapy is somewhat scarce among Asian Americans who suffer with trauma, some research has directed to the helpfulness of religious/ spiritual healing and well-being. For example, research has shown that among older Chinese and Korean Americans, religious coping strategies such as the practice of forgiveness, prayer, and meditation were associated with greater life satisfaction and self-efficacy, as well as decreased depression (Lee, 2007; Vilchinsky & Kravetz, 2005).

Specifically related to trauma and meaning making in psychotherapy, an investigation was conducted by Yeh et al. (2006) in which they interviewed 11 Asian Americans who had lost members of their families to the World Trade Center attacks on September 11, 2001. They examined the use of individualistic and collectivistic coping strategies among these Asian American family members who experienced this traumatic loss. The results indicated that Asian Americans utilized a spiritual collectivistic coping method to deal with their loss by believing in God, and as a result, was able to reintroduce meaning into their lives. Also, 4 of the 11 participants indicated that they increased their religious or spiritual activity by way of prayer, going to church, speaking with a pastor, and attending religious functions. These activities and beliefs may be connected to their interpretation and meaning of the loss, such as it "happened for a reason," or it "was in God's hands." It appears that spiritually oriented strategies not only assisted these Asian Americans in overcoming traumatic and distressful situations in life, but also helped them cope within their cultural context. When Esmeralda lost her son, she too began going to church, reconnecting with her congregation, and feeling God's love for her. These spiritually oriented strategies assisted Esmeralda to recreate meaning in her life.

Similarly, Heppner et al. (2006) found strong empirical support in a large quantitative study for both family support and religious/spiritual coping factors in East Asian individuals. Additional spiritually oriented practices for Asian American Christian believers are proposed. These practices include (1) prayer for the healing of the Holy Spirit offered at the beginning of the session, (2) relaxation exercises and Bible imagery, (3) directing the client to focus on the deep trauma and pain, (4) invoke the Lord to help heal through the Holy Spirit and minister His love and peace, (5) allow therapeutic silence as the client prayerfully waits to be ministered by the Lord, (6) end each session with prayer, and (7) debrief about inner healing that took place during session (Tan & Dong, 2014). Culturally sensitive psychotherapists who see clients of Asian descent may want to consider incorporating some of the above-mentioned spiritually oriented strategies in session.

Like many other racial, ethnic minorities in the United States where spirituality is deeply embedded in the fabric of their cultures, the amalgamation of culture and spirituality is not only salient, but also naturally infused in the everyday lives of American Indians and Alaska Natives. Owing to the diversity and variation of tribes among American Indians, it is a challenge to cover all of the spiritual uniqueness and values (Sue & Sue, 2012). However, below are various distilled cultural and spiritual values and strategies for psychotherapy from research conducted among American Indians. For more in-depth information about these strategies, we recommend that readers review these sources and references in more detail (Garrett & Portman, 2011; Garrett et al., 2011; Garrett & Wilbur, 1999; Garwick & Auger, 2003; King, Trimble, Morse, & Thomas, 2014; Trimble, 2010).

- Use of oral tradition of storytelling to teach each other and younger generations.
- Greeting circles, prayer, and burning of sage/sweetgrass to foster psychotherapist/client collectivity and honesty.
- Understanding and respecting the spiritual nature and value of each individual, animal, plant, and mineral (i.e., Mother Earth and Father Sky).
- Encouragement of dreams and visions for additional guidance.
- Seeking a traditional or spiritual healer.
- Sweat lodge for ceremonial purification.
- Utilization of extended family members for additional support in maintaining and rearing children and families.
- The value of the here-and-now aspect rather than preparation and time spent on future goals.
- The interconnection of spirit, mind, and body is essential when understanding illnesses.
- Listening is more valued than talking, and direct eye contact with an elder could be disrespectful.
- Recognition and respect for the higher power known as the Great One, Creator, Great Creator, or Great Spirit.

As psychotherapists work with American Indians, it is vital for them to first focus on being culturally sensitive before recognizing potential spiritual interventions that may help. As their culture and spirituality are intertwined into one, as you become culturally minded within their worldview lens (i.e., striving to remove biases, assumptions, prejudices about American Indians and their culture), spiritual pieces will follow naturally as potential interventions to incorporate into the session. For instance, psychotherapists should be aware that many American Indians adhere to the importance of sharing and giving among themselves and with others outside of their culture to maintain social harmony (Sue & Sue, 2012). They may want to share their gifts and other valuables with psychotherapists as a sign of respect and gratitude for services offered on their behalf. It is important for psychotherapists to recognize this as a cultural value and be sensitive to this respectful exchange.

Furthermore, American Indians and Alaska Natives had to endure a long history of traumatic exterminations and complicated efforts of assimilation (King et al., 2014). Due to protective factors like their strong spiritual and cultural aspects, strength and resilience for many were found through spirituality; spiritual connection to and respect for the earth and others; respect for traditional values; loyalty to family, tribe, and community; the values of the here-and-now (particularly related to possible efficacy of mindfulness in session); and personal attributes such as mastery, independence, and generosity (Gilgun, 2002; Sue & Sue, 2012). In addition, another strategy related to American Indian spirituality for psychotherapists is the importance of using spiritual language in session. Using language to normalize common Native beliefs is key. Suggestions could be utilizing the words *ceremonies* or *customs* rather than *rituals*. Similarly, *Creator* might be used rather than *God,* or *elder* in place of *mentor.* The goal is to implicitly (and explicitly) communicate respect for Native beliefs and willingness to work within the parameters of a Native understanding of reality (Hodge & Limb, 2010; King et al., 2014).

CLINICAL RECOMMENDATIONS FOR TRAUMA AND MEANING MAKING FOR RELIGIOUS ETHNIC MINORITIES IN THE UNITED STATES

The following section will provide basic foundational guidelines and recommendations when working with religious ethnic minorities in the United States who may be struggling with trauma. We do not contend that these are all encompassing solutions to every trauma case for each diverse group, but we do suggest that these can be helpful in establishing a culturally sensitive and oriented psychotherapy for ethnic diverse individuals in the United States.

Below are some of these recommendations:

- In some cases when working with someone who is culturally different from the psychotherapist, it can be beneficial to bring up the reality and also the reaction of the client to working with a psychotherapist of a different ethnic background. An example statement could be, "When clients are assigned to a therapist who is culturally different than the client, the client could feel uncomfortable about this? Is this something that may prevent us from working together?"

- Worldview, expectations, and values of the client are essential in assessing in the first session, particularly how these are related to their aims for psychotherapy. It would be wise to determine how the client perceives the trauma and potential remedies for meaning making.

- Many ethnic minorities may see the psychotherapist as an authority figure, it may be helpful to establish an egalitarian relationship with the client by (1) establishing a personal connection through exercising self-disclosure and (2) describing that typically psychotherapists are facilitators of healing who can help guide clients to improved mental health, but may not have all the answers and solutions clients seek.

- Investigating various culturally adapted and empirically supported psychotherapies may be discussed with ethnic minority clients. Potential solution-focused and problem solving may perhaps be preferred psychotherapies for trauma among religious ethnic minority individuals.

- Religious and spiritual interventions for trauma that are culturally specific should be discussed with ethnic minority clients early on in and throughout psychotherapy.

- Determine what positive resources are available to psychotherapy sessions, such as what are the social, familial, and environmental supports available for the clients? How have traumatic issues been positively dealt with in the past based on their cultural values?

- As there are many ethnic minority cultures that emphasize the body–mind connection, assess the severity of both traumatic struggles as well as physical symptoms due to the trauma.

- Be aware of family structure, dynamics, and the role that the family unit plays in the client's life. Seek to understand family roles of parents, grandparents, uncles, aunties, godfather, and godmother, as these family members could offer additional assistance with trauma through collaboration.

- Depending on how acculturation levels, sometimes a translator may be needed for both a language barrier and personal comfort with the native language when discussing potential intimate and private traumatic experiences.

CONCLUSIONS

Although we have provided some information related to efficacy and research of spiritually oriented psychotherapy strategies for trauma and meaning making, as well as its relevance to racial ethnic diverse individuals, there still remains more research and understanding needed to employ these strategies in the counseling session (Richards & Bergin, 2014). Additional training from experts and practitioners using these interventions with diverse populations in session would be helpful for psychotherapists who may want to incorporate spiritually oriented strategies with their clients. We hope that this chapter will stimulate interest of other educators, scholars, and researchers to advance the understanding and knowledge of spiritually oriented psychotherapy strategies for trauma among diverse populations.

Many lives affected with traumatic experiences, such as the loss of Esmeralda's son, thankfully, can be helped through hope and spiritual strategies. Frankl (1985), a concentration camp survivor during World War II, believed that life has meaning under all circumstances, even the most miserable ones. He contends that our main motivation for living is found in our will to find meaning in life. This opportunity to utilize spiritual methods to find meaning in what we do, and what we experience, or at least in the stand we take when faced with a situation of suffering, gives us hope and courage to continue.

REFERENCES

Ahrens, C. E., Abeling, S., Ahmad, S., & Hinman, J. (2010). Spirituality and well-being: the relationship between religious coping and recovery from sexual assault. *Journal of Interpersonal Violence, 25*(7), 1242–1263. http://dx.doi.org/10.1177/0886260509340533.

Allen, G. E., Garriott, P. O., Reyes, C. J., & Hsieh, C. (2013). Racial identity, phenotype, and self-esteem among biracial polynesian/white individuals. *Family Relations, 62*(1), 82–91.

Allen, G. E., & Heppner, P. P. (2011). Religiosity, coping, and psychological well-being among latter-day Saint Polynesians in the US. *Asian American Journal of Psychology, 2*(1), 13.

Allen, G. E. K., & Smith, T. (2015). Collectivistic coping strategies for distress among Polynesian Americans. *Psychological Services, 12*(3), 322.

Bernal, G., & Sáez-Santiago, E. (2006). Culturally centered psychosocial interventions. *Journal of Community Psychology, 34*(2), 121–132.

Berrett, M. E., Hardman, R. K., O'Grady, K. A., & Richards, P. S. (2007). The role of spirituality in the treatment of trauma and eating disorders: recommendations for clinical practice. *Eating Disorders: Journal of Treatment and Prevention, 15*, 373–389.

Blakley, T. L. (2007). The anatomy of trauma and faith: a reflective post-mortem. *Social Work & Christianity, 34*(1), 88–103.

Comas-Diaz, L. (2006). Latino healing: the integration of ethnic psychology into psychotherapy. *Psychotherapy: Theory, Research, Practice, Training, 43*(4), 436.

Conrad, M. M., & Pacquiao, D. F. (2005). Manifestation, attribution, and coping with depression among Asian Indians from the perspectives of health care practitioners. *Journal of Transcultural Nursing, 16*(1), 32–40.

Cook, D. A., & Wiley, C. Y. (2014). Psychotherapy with members of African American churches and spiritual traditions (pp. 373–397). In P. S. Richards, & A. E. Bergin (Eds.), *Handbook of psychotherapy and religious diversity* (2nd ed.). Washington, DC: American Psychological Association.

Frankl, V. E. (1985). *Man's search for meaning.* Simon and Schuster.

Frankl, V. E. (2006). *Man's search for meaning*. Boston: Beacon Press.

Gall, T. L. (2006). Spirituality and coping with life stress among adult survivors of childhood sexual abuse. *Child Abuse & Neglect, 30*(7), 829–844. http://dx.doi.org/10.1016/j.chiabu.2006.01.003.

Garrett, M. T., & Portman, T. A. A. (2011). *Counseling and diversity: Counseling native Americans*. Brooks/Cole.

Garrett, M. T., Torres-Rivera, E., Brubaker, M., Agahe Portman, T. A., Brotherton, D., West-Olatunji, C., … Grayshield, L. (2011). Crying for a vision: the native American sweat lodge ceremony as therapeutic intervention. *Journal of Counseling & Development, 89*(3), 318–325.

Garrett, M. T., & Wilbur, M. P. (1999). Does the worm live in the ground? Reflections on native American spirituality. *Journal of Multicultural Counseling and Development, 27*(4), 193–206.

Garwick, A. W., & Auger, S. (2003). Participatory action research: the Indian family stories project. *Nursing Outlook, 51*(6), 261–266.

Gilgun, J. F. (2002). Completing the circle: American Indian medicine wheels and the promotion of resilience of children and youth in care. *Journal of Human Behavior in the Social Environment, 6*(2), 65–84.

Grant, R. (1999). Spirituality and trauma: an essay. *Traumatology, 5*, 8–10.

Griner, D., & Smith, T. B. (2006). Culturally adapted mental health intervention: a meta-analytic review. *Psychotherapy: Theory, Research, Practice, Training, 43*(4), 531.

Grossman, F. K., Sorsoli, L., & Kia-Keating, M. (2006). A gale force wind: meaning making by male survivors of childhood sexual abuse. *American Journal of Orthopsychiatry, 76*(4), 434–443. http://dx.doi.org/10.1037/0002-9432.76.4.434.

Heppner, P. P., Heppner, M. J., Lee, D. G., Wang, Y. W., Park, H. J., & Wang, L. F. (2006). Development and validation of a collectivist coping styles inventory. *Journal of Counseling Psychology, 53*(1), 107.

Herman, J. L. (1992). *Trauma and recovery*. New York, NY, US: Basic Books.

Herman, J. L. (1997). *Trauma and recovery* (Vol. 551). New York, NY: Basic Books.

Hodge, D. R., & Limb, G. E. (2010). Conducting spiritual assessments with native Americans: enhancing cultural competency in social work practice courses. *Journal of Social Work Education, 46*(2), 265–284.

Holt, C. L., Lewellyn, L. A., & Rathweg, M. J. (2005). Exploring religion-health mediators among African American parishioners. *Journal of Health Psychology, 10*(4), 511–527.

Jacobson, C., Luckhaupt, S. E., Delaney, S., & Tsevat, J. (2006). Religio-biography, coping, and meaning-making among persons with HIV/AIDS. *Journal for the Scientific Study of Religion, 45*(1), 39–56.

King, J., Trimble, J. E., Morse, G. S., & Thomas, L. R. (2014). North American indian and Alaska native spirituality and psychotherapy (pp. 451–472). In P. S. Richards, & A. E. Bergin (Eds.), *Handbook of psychotherapy and religious diversity* (2nd ed.). Washington, DC: American Psychological Association.

Lee, E. K. O. (2007). Religion and spirituality as predictors of well-being among Chinese American and Korean American older adults. *Journal of Religion, Spirituality & Aging, 19*(3), 77–100.

McCubbin, L. D. (2006). Opinion Piece: indigenous values, cultural safety and improving health care: the case of native Hawaiians. *Contemporary Nurse, 22*(2), 214–217.

McCubbin, L. D., Ishikawa, M. E., & McCubbin, H. I. (2008). The Kanaka Maoli: native Hawaiians and their testimony of trauma and resilience. In *Ethnocultural perspectives on disaster and trauma (pp. 271–298)*. New York: Springer.

Parks, F. M., Zea, M. C., & Mason, M. A. (2014). Psychotherapy with members of Latino/Latina churches and spiritual traditions (pp. 399–421). In P. S. Richards, & A. E. Bergin (Eds.), *Handbook of psychotherapy and religious diversity* (2nd ed.). Washington, DC: American Psychological Association.

Pritt, A. F. (1998). Spiritual correlates of reported sexual abuse among Mormon women. *Journal for the Scientific Study of Religion, 37*(2), 273–285. http://dx.doi.org/10.2307/1387527.

Richards, P. S., & Bergin, A. E. (2004). *Casebook for a spiritual strategy in counseling and psychotherapy.* Washington, DC: American Psychological Association.

Richards, P. S., & Bergin, A. E. (2005). *A spiritual strategy for counseling and psychotherapy* (2nd ed.). Washington, DC: American Psychological Association.

Richards, P. S., & Bergin, A. E. (2014). *Handbook of psychotherapy and religious diversity* (2nd ed.). Washington, DC: American Psychological Association.

Richards, P. S., & Worthington, E. L., Jr. (2010). The need for evidence-based, spiritually oriented psychotherapies. *Professional Psychology: Research and Practice, 41*, 363–370.

Richardson, B. L., & June, L. N. (1997). Utilizing and maximizing the resources of the African American church: strategies and tools for counseling professionals. *Multicultural Issues in Counseling: New Approaches to Diversity, 2*, 155–170.

Ryan, P. L. (1998). An exploration of the spirituality of women who survived childhood violence. *Journal of Transpersonal Psychology, 30*(2), 87–102.

Seirmarco, G., Neria, Y., Insel, B., Kiper, D., Doruk, A., Gross, R., & Litz, B. (2012). Religiosity and mental health: changes in religious beliefs, complicated grief, posttraumatic stress disorder, and major depression following the September 11, 2001 attacks. *Psychology of Religion and Spirituality, 4*(1), 10–18. http://dx.doi.org/10.1037/a0023479.

Sperry, L., & Shafranske, E. P. (2005). *Spiritually oriented psychotherapy.* Washington, DC: American Psychological Association.

Sue, D. W., & Sue, D. (1999). *Counseling the culturally different: Theory and practice.*

Sue, D. W., & Sue, D. (2012). *Counseling the culturally diverse: Theory and practice.* John Wiley & Sons.

Tan, S. Y., & Dong, N. J. (2014). Psychotherapy with members of Asian American churches and spiritual traditions (pp. 423–450). In P. S. Richards, & A. E. Bergin (Eds.), *Handbook of psychotherapy and religious diversity* (2nd ed.). Washington, DC: American Psychological Association.

Trimble, J. E. (2010). Bear spends time in our dreams now: magical thinking and cultural empathy in multicultural counselling theory and practice. *Counseling Psychology Quarterly, 23*(3), 241–253.

Vilchinsky, N., & Kravetz, S. (2005). How are religious belief and behavior good for you? an investigation of mediators relating religion to mental health in a sample of Israeli Jewish students. *Journal for the Scientific Study of Religion, 44*(4), 459–471.

Walker, D. F., Courtois, C. A., & Aten, J. D. (2015). *Spiritually oriented psychotherapy for trauma.* Washington: American Psychological Association. http://dx.doi.org/10.1037/14500-000.

Weber, L. J., & Cummings, A. L. (2003). Relationships among spirituality, social support, and childhood maltreatment in university students. *Counseling and Values, 47*(2), 82–95. http://dx.doi.org/10.1002/j.2161-007X.2003.tb00226.x.

Yeh, C. J., Inman, A. C., Kim, A. B., & Okubo, Y. (2006). Asian American families' collectivistic coping strategies in response to 9/11. *Cultural Diversity & Ethnic Minority Psychology, 12*(1), 134–148.

Population Specific Applications

PART 3

Population Specific
Applications

CHAPTER 7

Reconstructing Meaning After Sexual Assault

P. Frazier, V. Nguyen-Feng, M. Baker

University of Minnesota, Minneapolis, MN, United States

CASE VIGNETTE

Emily was excited to begin her first year at Central State University. Although she was nervous about leaving her family and friends, she was comfortable at Central because she had often visited her brother there. She was also happy to see that the teaching assistant for one of her classes was a friend of her brother named Michael, whom she had met several times before.

One night Michael and Emily were at the same party and spent quite a bit of time hanging out. When the party was winding down, they were still having fun and Michael invited Emily back to his dorm room. Emily agreed because she trusted Michael. When they got to his room, they sat on the bed and talked and laughed some more. After a while, Michael started kissing Emily. She was enjoying the kissing but then Michael started to pull down her pants. She definitely did not want to have sex with Michael and told him so. He kept trying to talk her into it and telling her how turned on he was. She kept saying "No" and tried pushing him away. Michael was heavy on top of her and she could not get up. After more struggle, he penetrated her. Emily was eventually able to get up and sat for a while in shock. After about 30 min, Michael walked Emily back to her dorm room, and she went to bed without telling anyone what happened.

The next morning Emily's mind was reeling. On the one hand, she could not believe how stupid she had been. Why did she go to Michael's dorm room late at night? How many times had she been told not to go home with a guy from a party? Did she lead him on by letting him kiss her? Why had she not screamed or called for help? On the other hand, she could not figure out why he would do this to her. They were friends, he was friends with her brother, and she had trusted him. If she could not trust him, whom could she trust?

Reconstructing Meaning After Trauma
ISBN 978-0-12-803015-8
http://dx.doi.org/10.1016/B978-0-12-803015-8.00007-3

Over the next few weeks and months, Emily struggled in school. She had been doing well before but now she found it hard to concentrate. She blamed Michael for what he did but also blamed herself for letting it happen. She kept replaying the night over and over in her mind, wishing she had acted differently. Walking near Michael's dorm triggered more of these thoughts, so she found herself avoiding his dorm as well as all of her brother's friends. She could not sleep and felt tired and depressed. She often skipped class.

Her friends did not know what was going on and were starting to worry about her. She finally told them what had happened. Through talking with them, she started to see that it was not her fault. Although her friends were helpful, she decided that she did not want this event to ruin her college experience and that she needed to do everything she could to put it behind her. She made an appointment at the counseling center on campus.

Emily was nervous about going but was happy that she was assigned to a female counselor named Amy. She did not mention the assault at first but as she got to know Amy better she learned that Amy had recently completed an internship at a Veteran's Administration (VA) Medical Center where she received training in cognitive processing therapy (CPT) for posttraumatic stress disorder (PTSD). This gave Emily confidence that Amy would understand what she was going through and could help her deal with the assault. When Emily told Amy, she was both very understanding and very knowledgeable. Together, they worked through Emily's emotions and beliefs about the assault and what it meant to her life. Through this work Emily's symptoms of PTSD and depression decreased, and she also was able to come to terms with what had happened. Near the end of therapy, she decided to become an advocate for sexual assault survivors on campus and to use her experience to help others who have been through similar experiences.

CHAPTER OVERVIEW

Unfortunately, this fictional story of Emily and Michael is all too real. In the Association of American Universities (AAU) 2015 survey on sexual assault and sexual misconduct, almost 25% of undergraduate women reported nonconsensual sexual contact by physical force, threats of physical force, or incapacitation since entering college (AAU, 2015). Similarly, in the National Intimate Partner and Sexual Violence Survey, 18% of women in the United States reported having experienced a completed rape (Black et al., 2011).

Like Emily, most women are sexually assaulted by someone they knew (Black et al., 2011).

It is well established that sexual assault is associated with many mental health issues including depression, substance abuse, and PTSD (Walsh, Galea, & Koenen, 2012). In fact, rape is associated with a higher risk of PTSD than most other traumatic events, including combat (Kessler, Sonnega, Bromet, Hughes, & Nelson, 1995) and is one of the only lifetime events associated with current distress in college students (Frazier, Anders, et al., 2009). In addition, even though resilience (characterized by consistently low levels of symptoms) is the most common pattern following many traumatic events (Bonanno, 2004), there is some evidence that it is not the most common pattern following sexual assault (Steenkamp, Dickstein, Salters-Pedneault, Hofmann, & Litz, 2012). Indeed, nearly all survivors in Steenkamp et al.'s study reported high levels of distress 1 month postassault.

Although the reasons why sexual assault is so distressing are not entirely clear, it may be particularly distressing to experience a traumatic event involving intentional harm (Frazier, Anders, et al., 2009), especially by someone one trusts, like Emily trusted Michael. How can Emily make sense of this event? According to Park and George (2013), situational meaning (i.e., the meaning of a specific event versus broader beliefs about the meaning of one's life) involves processes related to trying to find meaning in an event (meaning making) as well as the outcomes of those processes (meaning(s) made). More specifically, Park and George described four different components of situational meaning: (1) the appraisal of an event (e.g., as controllable), (2) meaning-making processes (e.g., asking oneself "why" an event occurred), (3) appraisals of the extent to which an event violated one's global meaning (e.g., the belief that people can be trusted), and (4) meanings made (e.g., perceived positive life changes).

In this chapter, we review research on these components of situational meaning following sexual assault, linking them to Emily's experiences. We use this framework to lend some consistency to research in this area which often was not conceptualized in terms of meaning making (Park & George, 2013). Given space constraints, we cannot comprehensively review research on the myriad ways in which these components have been assessed. Rather, we will focus on the most common ways they have been assessed in research on sexual assault, citing representative studies. To limit the scope, we focus on adult sexual assault rather than child sexual abuse or other forms of interpersonal violence (IPV). We conclude with a discussion of interventions that address these meaning-making components.

EVENT APPRAISAL AND MEANING MAKING

One of Emily's first reactions to the assault was to question whether she was to blame. Studies of women who have recently been assaulted have suggested that self-blame is common (e.g., Frazier, 2000, 2003). Feminist theory contends that the larger context of a "culture of blame" around sexual assault facilitates the notion that the rape was somehow the survivor's fault (McKenzie-Mohr, 2014). Research showing that self-blame was more common in sexual assault survivors compared with survivors of other traumas (e.g., Moor & Farchi, 2011) lends credence to the notion that sexual assault survivors wrestle with self-blame when searching for meaning in ways that other survivors may not.

Unfortunately, studies show that survivors who engaged in more self-blame tended to report more distress (e.g., Frazier, 2003) and were at increased risk for revictimization (e.g., Katz, May, Sorensen, & DelTosta, 2010). The appraisal that the assault was controllable also was associated with more distress (e.g., Frazier, 2000). Importantly, survivors who reported blaming the assailant and blaming society were also more distressed (Frazier, 2000, 2003).

These findings led to the development of a new model of control appraisals (Frazier, 2003; Frazier et al., 2011) that focuses on the distinctions between past control (including attributions regarding why the assault occurred), present control (e.g., control over the recovery process), and future control (e.g., control over being assaulted again). In a longitudinal study of recent sexual assault survivors, the only control appraisal that was associated with less distress was perceived control over the recovery process, an aspect of present control (Frazier, 2003; see also Ullman, Filipas, Townsend, & Starzynski, 2007). Unlike past or future assaults, the recovery process is an aspect of the assault that can actually be controlled. For Emily, talking to her friends helped her to stop blaming herself and focus more on her recovery process, consistent with research findings (e.g., Frazier, Mortensen, & Steward, 2005).

Relatively little research has focused on the meaning-making process following sexual assault. In our work, we have found that survivors who reported thinking more often about "why" the rape occurred were more distressed (Frazier, 2000). This may be because they may still be trying to make sense of the event. Two small qualitative studies (Harvey, Orbuch, Chwalisz, & Garwood, 1991; Orbuch, Harvey, Davis, & Merbachet, 1994) found that engaging in more account making (i.e., constructing stories of events that include explanations) and completeness of account making were associated with better adjustment among assault survivors. In the Orbuch et al. study, which included both open-ended and structured questions, some participants mentioned that responses to structured questions did not reflect the complexity of their experiences, suggesting that qualitative research may be useful for understanding the meaning–making process.

VIOLATIONS OF GLOBAL MEANING

Another component of Park and George's (2013) meaning making model involves an appraisal of the extent to which events violate basic assumptions about the self and world. It is often assumed that traumatic events "shatter" positive pretrauma assumptions (e.g., that the world is safe). For example, after being assaulted by Michael, Emily felt much less trusting than she had before.

The best way to determine whether traumatic events actually change basic assumptions is to assess assumptions before and after a traumatic event. This is difficult because we do not know in advance who will experience a trauma. One small study attempted to address this issue by comparing changes in assumptions among survivors of physical intimate partner violence who had or had not experienced interpersonal revictimization 1 year later (Valdez & Lilly, 2015). If traumatic events shatter assumptions, those who were revictimized should report more negative changes in assumptions than those who were not revictimized. However, world assumptions became more positive in the absence of revictimization but were unchanged in survivors who were revictimized. Thus, assumptions did not necessarily worsen with more exposure to trauma.

More often, studies assess whether sexual assault is associated with belief change by comparing individuals with and without a history of sexual assault on measures of assumptions. Studies using this method have produced mixed results, although victims have consistently reported lower self-worth (e.g., Harris & Valentiner, 2002; Littleton, Grills-Taquechel, Axsom, Bye, & Buck, 2012). However, these data do not necessarily support the conclusion that assumptions changed from pre- to postassault. We cannot assume that individuals who have been assaulted as adults had positive beliefs about themselves and the world before the assault, especially given the frequency with which adult victims were also victimized as children (Gilfus, 1999). It is clear, however, that survivors who had more negative beliefs about themselves and the world reported more distress (e.g., Harris & Valentiner, 2002; Littleton et al., 2012).

Another way to assess whether a traumatic event has shattered assumptions is to directly ask survivors whether their beliefs have changed. In one study, 60–83% of recent sexual assault survivors reported that their beliefs about the goodness of people and the safety and fairness of the world had changed for the worse as a result of the assault (Frazier, Conlon, & Glaser, 2001). In another sample of women who had been sexually assaulted several years previously, 32–48% reported negative changes in these beliefs (Frazier, Conlon, Steger, Tashiro, & Glaser, 2006). Other studies have found that almost all survivors reported negative beliefs about trust (Fairbrother & Rachman, 2006) and 20–48% reported becoming less religious (Ben-Ezra et al., 2010; Kennedy, Davis, & Taylor, 1998).

POSTTRAUMATIC GROWTH: POSITIVE MEANING MADE

Although traumatic events such as sexual assault may negatively affect one's assumptions about the world, survivors often create positive meanings out of traumatic events. In fact, one of the most common ways in which "meaning made" has been assessed is through measures of self-reported growth (Park & George, 2013). Our work in this area began before the development of structured measures of posttraumatic growth. In our first study, we asked recent sexual assault survivors whether the assault had caused any positive changes in their lives (Frazier & Burnett, 1994). Just 3 days postassault, 57% reported some positive change. Of the nine categories reported, the most common was that they were now more cautious (see also Draucker, 2001).

Based on these initial data, we developed a more structured measure of positive (and negative) life changes following sexual assault that assessed changes in self, spirituality/life philosophy, relationships, and empathy (Frazier et al., 2001). At 2 weeks postassault, 91% of a sample of sexual assault survivors reported at least one positive change resulting from the assault. Greater empathy (more concern for others in similar situations) was the most common positive change reported across four time points from 2 weeks to 1 year postassault. This was also the most common positive change reported in a community sample of women who had been assaulted several years previously (Frazier et al., 2006). In another study, 60% of sexual assault survivors reported increased spirituality (Kennedy et al., 1998).

Now, the most commonly used measure of self-reported growth is the Posttraumatic Growth Inventory (PTGI; Tedeschi & Calhoun, 1996). The PTGI asks individuals to retrospectively report the extent to which their life has changed in a positive manner in five domains (e.g., appreciation of life, new possibilities) as the result of a traumatic event. Studies using this measure reveal that, similar to other traumatic events, many survivors (e.g., 74–100%) reported positive life changes following sexual assault (e.g., Ahrens, Abeling, Ahmad, & Hinman, 2010; Cole & Lynn, 2010).

Because the PTGI does not assess increased compassion or altruism following trauma, this area of potential growth has been neglected in the literature (Frazier et al., 2013). However, as mentioned, greater compassion was the most commonly reported positive change in two samples of sexual assault survivors (Frazier et al., 2001, 2006). Similarly, in a qualitative study of survivors of sexual violence (including child abuse and adult sexual assault), 69% spontaneously mentioned helping others as a way of healing (Stidham, Draucker, Martsolf, & Mullen, 2012). An analysis of these responses revealed nine different ways of helping others, including choosing a helping profession, providing advocacy, and speaking publicly. According to the authors, the participants in their study emphasized that helping others helped them make sense of their experiences and reflected their desire to have something good come from their pain. Emily's decision to become an advocate for sexual assault survivors on campus illustrates the potential role of helping others in the healing process.

As was mentioned in the section on changes in assumptions, the best way to assess whether individuals have actually grown as the result of a sexual assault or other traumatic event is to assess domains of potential growth before and after a trauma. We are aware of no studies that have used this prospective design to assess growth from before to after a sexual assault, and such studies are rare in the trauma field in general. One study that used a prospective design found that the correlations between perceived growth (assessed using the PTGI) and "actual" growth [assessed via increases in measures reflecting the PTGI domains (e.g., life appreciation) from pre- to posttrauma] revealed very small correlations between the measures of perceived and actual growth, suggesting that self-reported positive changes may not always be veridical (Frazier, Tennen, et al., 2009). Moreover, perceived growth was associated with more distress, whereas actual growth was associated with less distress. Perceived, but not actual, growth was strongly associated with positive reappraisal coping, suggesting that reporting positive changes may be a way of coping with distress (see also Gunty et al., 2011).

In summary, retrospective reports of positive or negative life changes as a result of a sexual assault cannot necessarily be assumed to reflect actual change from pre- to postassault. Positive meanings made also cannot be assumed to be associated with less distress or better adjustment. In studies of sexual assault survivors, the relations between measures of growth and distress have been mixed (Frazier & Berman, 2008).

INTERVENTIONS ADDRESSING MEANING MAKING

This review has revealed several findings that have been replicated across studies. First, self-blame is consistently associated with more distress, whereas focusing on what can be controlled in the present (such as the recovery process) is consistently associated with less distress. Second, survivors often report that their beliefs changed in a negative direction following an assault and having more negative beliefs is associated with reporting more distress. Finally, survivors often report positive life changes, particularly more compassion for others. In the concluding section, we discuss research on interventions for sexual assault that address these components of meaning making.

CPT was developed specifically to treat PTSD in sexual assault survivors (Resick & Schnicke, 1992). It has since been adapted to treat PTSD following other traumas and is one of the few empirically supported PTSD treatments disseminated by the VA. CPT is designed to help survivors both to reduce their fear (through exposure) and to change their beliefs about and the meaning of the event (through cognitive techniques). The cognitive component includes training in identifying thoughts and feelings, and techniques for challenging maladaptive beliefs regarding safety, trust, power, esteem, and intimacy. At the beginning and end of CPT, survivors write impact statements in which they write about the meaning of the event.

Several studies support the efficacy of CPT in reducing distress following sexual assault. In the first randomized controlled trial (RCT), those in the CPT condition reported greater reductions in distress than those in a wait-list group (Resick, 1992). Subsequent studies have shown that CPT is as effective as prolonged exposure (PE) and better than minimal attention in reducing symptoms, that CPT was somewhat more effective than PE in reducing guilt (Resick, Nishith, Weaver, Astin, & Feuer, 2002), and that treatment gains were maintained 5–10 years later (Resick, Williams, Suvak, Monson, & Gradus, 2012). Analyses of the impact statements from the original RCT showed that accommodated thinking (i.e., balanced, accurate evaluations of self, others, and the world) increased and overaccommodated thinking (i.e., inaccurate overgeneralizations about self, others, and the world) decreased following treatment (Sobel, Resick, & Rabalais, 2009), and that these changes were maintained 5–10 years later (Iverson, King, Cunningham, & Resick, 2015). In addition, increases in accommodated thinking and decreases in overaccommodated thinking were associated with decreases in PTSD and depression symptoms over time (Iverson et al., 2015; Sobel et al., 2009). Changes in cognitions have also been found to mediate decreases in PTSD symptoms following PE (e.g., McLean, Yeh, Rosenfield, & Foa, 2015).

Based on the finding that perceived present control, including perceived control over the recovery process, is consistently associated with less distress, our research group developed a brief intervention designed to help individuals focus on what they can control in the present (rather than focusing on what they could have done in the past). We designed this as an internet-based intervention to reduce some of the barriers to accessing traditional mental health services such as stigma and time constraints. Our first RCTs tested the efficacy of our intervention in general samples of college students and found that it was effective in reducing symptoms of stress, anxiety, and depression and that increases in present control mediated decreases in symptoms (Frazier et al., 2015; Hintz, Frazier, & Meredith, 2015). In a subsequent study, we found that our intervention was more effective for students exposed to IPV, including sexual assault, than for those not exposed (Nguyen-Feng et al., 2015). Rather than offering a trauma-focused intervention specifically to students with an IPV history, we were able to reach those students by offering a general stress management intervention to a large group of students, 39% of whom had an IPV history.

We found no research assessing whether promoting social action is helpful in the sexual assault recovery process, although some research has addressed this topic with cancer patients with mixed results. One intervention study with cancer survivors found that helping others reduced distress and improved health-related quality of life (Rini et al., 2014), whereas another found that breast cancer survivors assigned to an intervention in which they helped others reported more distress postintervention (Lepore et al., 2014). Thus, even though some authors encourage social action as a means of healing for sexual assault survivors (McKenzie-Mohr, 2014), research is needed to assess the efficacy of such interventions, especially since volunteer trauma workers with nonresolved traumas may be at risk for experiencing more distress than those with resolved traumas (Hargrave, Scott, & McDowall, 2006).

CONCLUSIONS AND CLINICAL IMPLICATIONS

We conclude with several implications for practitioners of the research we reviewed. Note that we do not say practitioners working with sexual violence survivors because many practitioners are likely to work with individuals who have survived some form of sexual violence but have not self-disclosed it.

Thus, our first suggestion is for practitioners to ask clients about their trauma history. Most individuals have experienced traumatic events in their lifetimes (Kessler et al., 1995) and, as noted previously, about 20% of women have experienced a completed rape (Black et al., 2011). Recent evidence suggests that many of these events may not be disclosed in therapy. For example, Rossiter et al. (2015) found that childhood trauma rates were much higher (77%) when clients completed a structured questionnaire than rates documented in clinical notes (38%) in a mental health clinic. For child sexual abuse in particular, 25% of clients reported this form of trauma on a questionnaire, whereas it was documented in only 9% of clinical notes. We are not aware of similar research assessing the discrepancy between standard questionnaires and clinical notes in terms of documenting adult sexual assault experiences but the discrepancy is likely there as well. There are several standard measures of trauma exposure such as the Trauma Life Events Questionnaire (Kubany et al., 2000) that can be used in practice. See the National Center for PTSD Website for more information (www.ptsd.va.gov/professional/assessment/te-measures/chart-trauma-exposure.asp).

Other suggestions apply to practitioners working with individuals who they know have experienced sexual violence. Even if this is not the client's presenting issue, practitioners might want to assess areas known to be affected by sexual violence (e.g., interpersonal relationships). The Trauma Symptom Inventory (Briere, 1995) is one well-known measure that assesses a range of posttrauma issues beyond PTSD symptoms. Again, the National Center for PTSD website has more information on trauma symptom measures, many of which focus specifically on PTSD (www.ptsd.va.gov/professional/assessment/adult-sr/chart-adult-self-report.asp). Our research shows that, among college students like Emily, sexual victimization is also related to poorer academic performance and risk of dropout (Baker et al., 2016). This is an additional domain that should be assessed with college students.

Most relevant to this chapter are specific suggestions for working with sexual violence as a clinical issue and in particular working with issues related to meaning making. We have reviewed evidence suggesting that self-blame and negative changes in beliefs are associated with more distress, whereas focusing on what can be controlled in the present is associated with less distress. In addition to assessing these issues clinically during the course of therapy, there are standard assessment instruments that can be used to assess these issues more systematically. For example, the Posttraumatic Cognitions Inventory (Foa, Ehlers, Clark, Tolin, & Orsillo, 1999) has subscales assessing Negative Cognitions About Self, Negative Cognitions About the World, and Self-Blame. The Perceived Control Over Stressful Events Scale (PCOSES; Frazier et al., 2011, 2012) assesses past, present, and future control over stressful life events and the perceived likelihood of similar events occurring again. The PCOSES can be used in reference to a specific event such as a sexual assault. As mentioned, the PTGI (Tedeschi & Calhoun, 1996) is the most commonly used measure of self-reported posttraumatic growth, although other measures have been developed specifically to assess positive and negative life changes following sexual assault (see Frazier et al., 2001).

We noted earlier that CPT is an empirically supported treatment for PTSD following sexual trauma with several studies supporting its efficacy. A web-based training program in CPT is freely available online along with worksheets and other clinical tools (https://cpt.musc.edu). We encourage practitioners working with survivors to avail themselves of these resources.

REFERENCES

AAU. (2015). Retrieved from: http://discover.umn.edu/sites/default/files/University%20of%20Minnesota%20-%20Twin%20Cities_9.21.15_%20Report.pdf.

Ahrens, C. E., Abeling, S., Ahmad, S., & Hinman, J. (2010). Spirituality and well-being: the relationship between religious coping and recovery from sexual assault. *Journal of Interpersonal Violence, 25,* 1242–1263. http://dx.doi.org/10.1177/0886260509340533.

Baker, M. R., Frazier, P. A., Greer, C., Paulsen, J. A., Howard, K., Meredith, L. N., Anders, S. L., & Shallcross, S. L. (February 25, 2016). Sexual victimization history predicts academic performance in college women. *Journal of Counseling Psychology.* Advance online publication. http://dx.doi.org/10.1037/cou0000146.

Ben-Ezra, M., Palgi, Y., Sternberg, D., Berkley, H., Glidai, Y., Moshe, L., & Shrira, A. (2010). Losing my religion: a preliminary study of changes. *Traumatology, 16,* 7–13. http://dx.doi.org/10.1177/1534765609358465.

Black, M. C., Basile, K. C., Breiding, M. J., Smith, S. G., Walters, M. L., Merrick, M. T., … Stevens, M. R. (2011). *The National Intimate Partner and Sexual Violence Survey (NISVS): 2010 summary report.* Atlanta, GA: National Center for Injury Prevention and Control, Centers for Disease Control and Prevention.

Bonanno, G. A. (2004). Loss, trauma, and human resilience: have we underestimated the human capacity to thrive after extremely aversive events? *American Psychologist, 59,* 20–28. http://dx.doi.org/10.1037/0003-066X.59.1.20.

Briere, J. (1995). *Trauma Symptom Inventory (TSI) professional manual.* Odessa, Florida: Psychological Assessment Resources.

Cole, A. S., & Lynn, S. J. (2010). Adjustment of sexual assault survivors: hardiness and acceptance coping in posttraumatic growth. *Imagination, Cognition, and Personality, 30,* 111–127.

Draucker, C. B. (2001). Learning the harsh realities of life: sexual violence, disillusionment, and meaning. *Health Care for Women International, 22,* 67–84. http://dx.doi.org/10.1080/073993301300003081.

Fairbrother, N., & Rachman, S. (2006). PTSD in victims of sexual assault: test of a major component of the Ehlers–Clark theory. *Journal of Behavior Therapy and Experimental Psychiatry, 37,* 74–93. http://dx.doi.org/10.1016/j.jbtep.2004.08.004.

Foa, E. B., Ehlers, A., Clark, D. M., Tolin, D. F., & Orsillo, S. M. (1999). The posttraumatic cognitions inventory (PTCI): development and validation. *Psychological Assessment, 11,* 303–314. http://dx.doi.org/10.1037/1040-3590.11.3.303.

Frazier, P. A. (2000). The role of attributions and perceived control in recovery from rape. *Journal of Personal and Interpersonal Loss, 5,* 203–225. http://dx.doi.org/10.1080/10811440008409753. Reprinted in J.H. Harvey and B.G. Pauwels (Eds.), *Posttraumatic Stress Theory, Research, and Application.* Philadelphia: Bruner/Mazel.

Frazier, P. A. (2003). Perceived control and distress following sexual assault: a longitudinal test of a new model. *Journal of Personality and Social Psychology, 84,* 1257–1269. http://dx.doi.org/10.1037/0022-3514.84.6.1257.

Frazier, P. A., Anders, S., Perera, S., Tomich, P., Tennen, H., Park, C., & Tashiro, T. (2009). Traumatic events among undergraduate students: prevalence and associated symptoms. *Journal of Counseling Psychology, 56,* 450–460. http://dx.doi.org/10.1037/a0016412.

Frazier, P. A., Anders, S., Shallcross, S., Keenan, N., Perera, S., Howard, K., & Hintz, S. (2012). Further development of the temporal model of control. *Journal of Counseling Psychology, 59,* 623–630. http://dx.doi.org/10.1037/a0029702.

Frazier, P., & Berman, M. (2008). Posttraumatic growth following sexual assault. In S. Joseph, & P. Alex Linley (Eds.), *Trauma, recovery, and growth: Positive psychological perspectives on posttraumatic stress* (pp. 161–181). Hoboken, NJ: John Wiley and Sons.

Frazier, P. A., & Burnett, J. (1994). Immediate coping strategies among rape victims. *Journal of Counseling and Development, 72,* 633–639. http://dx.doi.org/10.1002/j.1556-6676.1994.tb01694.x.

Frazier, P. A., Conlon, A., & Glaser, T. (2001). Positive and negative life changes following sexual assault. *Journal of Consulting and Clinical Psychology, 69,* 1048–1055. http://dx.doi.org/10.1037/AJ022-006X.69.6.1048.

Frazier, P., Conlon, A., Steger, M., Tashiro, T., & Glaser, T. (2006). Positive life changes following sexual assault: A replication and extension. In F. Columbo (Ed.), *Post-traumatic Stress: New Research* (pp. 1–22). Hauppauge, NY: Nova Science Publishers.

Frazier, P. A., Greer, C., Gabrielsen, S., Tennen, H., Park, C., & Tomich, P. (2013). The relation between trauma exposure and prosocial behavior. *Psychological Trauma: Theory, Research, Practice, and Policy, 5,* 286–294. http://dx.doi.org/10.1037/a0027255.

Frazier, P. A., Keenan, N., Anders, S., Perera, S., Shallcross, S., & Hintz, S. (2011). Perceived past, present, and future control and adjustment to stressful life events. *Journal of Personality and Social Psychology, 100,* 749–765. http://dx.doi.org/10.1037/a0022405.

Frazier, P. A., Meredith, L., Greer, C., Paulsen, J. A., Howard, K., Dietz, L., & Qin, K. (2015). Randomized controlled trial evaluating the effectiveness of a web-based stress management program among community college students. *Anxiety, Stress, and Coping, 28,* 576–586. http://dx.doi.org/10.1080/10615806.2014.987666.

Frazier, P. A., Mortensen, H., & Steward, J. (2005). Coping strategies as mediators of the relations among perceived control and distress in sexual assault survivors. *Journal of Counseling Psychology, 52,* 267–278. http://dx.doi.org/10.1037/0022-0167.52.3.267.

Frazier, P. A., Tennen, H., Gavian, M., Park, C., Tomich, P., & Tashiro, T. (2009). Does self-reported post-traumatic growth reflect genuine positive change? *Psychological Science, 20,* 912–919. http://dx.doi.org/10.1111/j.1467-9280.2009.02381.x.

Gilfus, M. E. (1999). The price of the ticket: a survivor-centered appraisal of trauma theory. *Violence Against Women, 5,* 1238–1257. http://dx.doi.org/10.1177/1077801299005011002.

Gunty, A., Frazier, P. A., Tennen, H., Tomich, P., Tashiro, T., & Park, C. (2011). Moderators of the relation between perceived and actual posttraumatic growth. *Psychological Trauma: Theory, Research, Practice, and Policy, 3,* 61–66. http://dx.doi.org/10.1037/a0020485.

Hargrave, P. A., Scott, K. M., & McDowall, J. (2006). To resolve or not to resolve: past trauma and secondary traumatic stress in volunteer crisis workers. *Journal of Trauma Practice, 5,* 37–55. http://dx.doi.org/10.1300/J189v05n02_03.

Harris, H. N., & Valentiner, D. P. (2002). World assumptions, sexual assault, depression, and fearful attitudes toward relationships. *Journal of Interpersonal Violence, 17,* 286–305. http://dx.doi.org/10.1177/0886260502017003004.

Harvey, J. H., Orbuch, T. L., Chwalisz, K. D., & Garwood, G. (1991). Coping with sexual assault: the roles of account-making and confiding. *Journal of Traumatic Stress, 4,* 515–531. http://dx.doi.org/10.1007/BF00974587.

Hintz, S., Frazier, P. A., & Meredith, L. (2015). Evaluating an online stress management intervention for college students. *Journal of Counseling Psychology, 62,* 137–147. http://dx.doi.org/10.1037/cou0000014.

Iverson, K. M., King, M. W., Cunningham, K. C., & Resick, P. A. (2015). Rape survivors' trauma-related beliefs before and after cognitive processing therapy: associations with PTSD and depression symptoms. *Behaviour Research and Therapy, 66,* 49–55.

Katz, J., May, P., Sorensen, S., & DelTosta, J. (2010). Sexual revictimization during women's first year of college: self-blame and sexual refusal assertiveness as possible mechanisms. *Journal of Interpersonal Violence, 25,* 2113–2126. http://dx.doi.org/10.1177/0886260509354515.

Kennedy, J. E., Davis, R. C., & Taylor, B. G. (1998). Changes in spirituality and well-being among victims of sexual assault. *Journal for the Scientific Study of Religion, 37,* 322–328. http://dx.doi.org/10.2307/1387531.

Kessler, R. C., Sonnega, A., Bromet, E., Hughes, M., & Nelson, C. B. (1995). Posttraumatic stress disorder in the national comorbidity survey. *JAMA Psychiatry, 52,* 1048–1060. http://dx.doi.org/10.1001/archpsyc.1995.03950240066012.

Kubany, E. S., Leisen, M. B., Kaplan, A. S., Watson, S. B., Haynes, S. N., Owens, J. A., & Burns, K. (2000). Development and preliminary validation of a brief broad-spectrum measure of trauma exposure: the traumatic life events questionnaire. *Psychological Assessment, 12,* 210–224. http://dx.doi.org/10.1037/1040-3590.12.2.210.

Lepore, S. J., Buzaglo, J. S., Lieberman, M., Golant, M., Greener, J., & Davey, A. (2014). Comparing standard versus prosocial internet support groups for patients with breast cancer: a randomized controlled trial of the helper therapy principle. *Journal of Clinical Oncology, 32,* 4081–4086. http://dx.doi.org/10.1200/JCO.2014.57.0093.

Littleton, H. L., Grills-Taquechel, A. E., Axsom, D., Bye, K., & Buck, K. S. (2012). Prior sexual trauma and adjustment following the Virginia tech campus shootings: examination of the mediating role of schemas and social support. *Psychological Trauma: Theory, Research, Practice, and Policy, 4,* 578–586. http://dx.doi.org/10.1037/a0025270.

McKenzie-Mohr, S. (2014). Counter-storying rape: women's efforts towards liberatory meaning making. In S. McKenzie-Mohr, & M. N. Lafrance (Eds.), *Women voicing resistance: Discursive and narrative explorations* (pp. 64–83). New York, NY: Routledge.

McLean, C. P., Yeh, R., Rosenfield, D., & Foa, E. B. (2015). Changes in negative cognitions mediate PTSD symptom reductions during client-centered therapy and prolonged exposure for adolescents. *Behaviour Research and Therapy, 68,* 64–69.

Moor, A., & Farchi, M. (2011). Is rape-related self-blame distinct from other post traumatic attributions of blame? A comparison of severity and implications for treatment. *Women and Therapy, 34,* 447–460. http://dx.doi.org/10.1080/02703149.2011.591671.

Nguyen-Feng, V. N., Frazier, P. A., Greer, C. S., Howard, K. G., Paulsen, J. A., Meredith, L., & Kim, S. (2015). A randomized controlled trial of a web-based intervention to reduce distress among students with a history of interpersonal violence. *Psychology of Violence, 5,* 444–454. http://dx.doi.org/10.1037/a0039596 Online first publication.

Orbuch, T. L., Harvey, J. H., Davis, S. H., & Merbach, N. J. (1994). Account-making and confiding as acts of meaning in response to sexual assault. *Journal of Family Violence, 9,* 249–264.

Park, C. L., & George, L. S. (2013). Assessing meaning and meaning making in the context of stressful life events: measurement tools and approaches. *Journal of Positive Psychology, 8,* 483–504. http://dx.doi.org/10.1080/17439760.2013.830762.

Resick, P. A., Nishith, P., Weaver, T. L., Astin, M. C., & Feuer, C. A. (2002). A comparison of cognitive-processing therapy with prolonged exposure and a waiting condition for the treatment of chronic posttraumatic stress disorder in female rape victims. *Journal of Consulting and Clinical Psychology, 70,* 867–879.

Resick, P. A., & Schnicke, M. K. (1992). Cognitive processing therapy for sexual assault victims. *Journal of Consulting and Clinical Psychology, 60,* 748–756.

Resick, P. A., Williams, L. F., Suvak, M. K., Monson, C. M., & Gradus, J. L. (2012). Long term outcomes of cognitive behavioral treatments for posttraumatic stress disorder among female rape survivors. *Journal of Consulting and Clinical Psychology, 80,* 201–210. http://dx.doi.org/10.1037/a0026602.

Rini, C., Austin, J., Wu, L. M., Winkel, G., Valdimarsdottir, H., Stanton, A. L., ... Redd, W. H. (2014). Harnessing benefits of helping others: a randomized controlled trial testing expressive helping to address survivorship problems after hematopoietic stem cell transplant. *Health Psychology, 33,* 1541–1551.

Rossiter, A., Byrne, F., Wota, A. P., Nisar, Z., Ofuafor, T., Murray, I., ... Hallahan, B. (2015). Childhood trauma levels in individuals attending adult mental health services: an evaluation of clinical records and structured measurement of childhood trauma. *Child Abuse & Neglect, 44,* 36–45. http://dx.doi.org/10.1016/j.chiabu.2015.01.001.

Sobel, A. A., Resick, P. A., & Rabalais, A. E. (2009). The effect of cognitive processing therapy on cognitions: impact statement coding. *Journal of Traumatic Stress, 22,* 205–211.

Steenkamp, M. M., Dickstein, B. D., Salters-Pedneault, K., Hofmann, S. G., & Litz, B. T. (2012). Trajectories of PTSD symptoms following sexual assault: is resilience the modal outcome? *Journal of Traumatic Stress, 25,* 469–474. http://dx.doi.org/10.1002/jts.21718.

Stidham, A. W., Martsolf, D. S., Draucker, C. B., & Mullen, L. P. (2012). Altruism in survivors of sexual violence: the typology of helping others. *Journal of the American Psychiatric Nurses Association, 18,* 146–155. http://dx.doi.org/10.1177/1078390312440595.

Tedeschi, R. G., & Calhoun, L. G. (1996). The posttraumatic growth inventory: measuring the positive legacy of trauma. *Journal of Traumatic Stress, 9,* 455–471. http://dx.doi.org/10.1007/BF02103658.

Ullman, S. E., Filipas, H. H., Townsend, S. M., & Starzynski, L. L. (2007). Psychosocial correlates of PTSD symptom severity in sexual assault survivors. *Journal of Traumatic Stress, 20,* 821–831.

Valdez, C. E., & Lilly, M. M. (2015). Posttraumatic growth in survivors of intimate partner violence: an assumptive world process. *Journal of Interpersonal Violence, 30,* 215–231. http://dx.doi.org/10.1177/0886260514533154.

Walsh, K., Galea, S., & Koenen, K. C. (2012). Mechanisms underlying sexual violence exposure and psychosocial sequelae: a theoretical and empirical review. *Clinical Psychology: Science and Practice, 19,* 260–275. http://dx.doi.org/10.1111/cpsp.12004.

CHAPTER 8

Growth and Meaning From Negotiating the Complex Journey of Being an Emergency Medical Dispatcher

J. Shakespeare-Finch[1], K. Adams[2]

[1]Queensland University of Technology, Brisbane, QLD, Australia; [2]Caboolture Regional Domestic Violence Service, Caboolture, QLD, Australia

JULIA

Julia works as an emergency medical dispatcher (EMD). Among the many difficulties Julia has faced in her role was the death of a close colleague and friend. Bob was a young man who had been in the organization only for about 2 years but he and Julia had become friends almost immediately. In fact, the EMD team felt like a family. They always had a catch-up and chat before each shift and had the usual conflicts families have as well as the fun and laughter. Their shared experiences created a bond between them—after all, not many people could really understand what a work day was like for them. Bob had recently broken up with his girlfriend. They had been high school sweethearts and Bob had assumed they would marry, have children, and spend the rest of their lives together. However, things changed after school and as they both finished their training and entered the workforce, his girlfriend had decided that she wanted to experience more of the world and learn more about herself as an individual so she had ended their relationship. Julia and Bob had spoken about how difficult the breakup was but Bob assured her he was okay and understood the reasons his girlfriend had made her decision. They would remain friends. What Julia and the rest of the team did not know was that Bob had been battling with a mental health issue for most of his adolescence and now, in his early 20s, the breakup had hit him hard. Julia recounts that he had worn a "mask" in the workplace to hide his distress. Suddenly Bob committed suicide. Julia was left traumatized by this experience. The organization Julia works for has a comprehensive system of staff support and counselors were immediately deployed to their

Reconstructing Meaning After Trauma
ISBN 978-0-12-803015-8
http://dx.doi.org/10.1016/B978-0-12-803015-8.00008-5

117

work place. One of the counselors stayed for a week, just to be around if people wanted to talk. As Julia tried to come to terms with Bob's suicide, she decided to have a talk with the counselor. They are still talking.

Help is only a phone call away. We memorize our national emergency phone number as early as childhood to hold close for times when things may go wrong. When we call, few would pause to consider the emotional impacts their own traumatic experience may have on the disembodied voice that answers that initial call and dispatches help and advice. There is often very little identity placed on that very first helper via telecommunications. In today's global and digital age, initial responses to crisis can be dealt with more immediately via remote services, including phone line or live web connections. For medical crisis, the unseen role of the EMD has historically been seemingly unrecognized both in literature and the public eye. But new research is emerging that shines light on the personal impacts for those who provide the first response remotely in an emergency (Adams, Shakespeare-Finch, & Armstrong, 2014; Shakespeare-Finch, Rees, & Armstrong, 2014).

To narrate this journey you are introduced to Julia. Julia is a real person, but her anonymity has been protected. The quotes that are in this chapter are accurately taken from a transcribed interview. Following an introduction to Julia and a description of the role that she holds, examples of the relatively high levels of exposure to stressful and potentially traumatic events she has faced are outlined. Organizational and operational factors that challenge her mental health are presented in her own words. The chapter then links Julia's story to research in this area and, interspersed with quotes from her interview, the chapter unpacks how she copes with and makes sense of the difficulties inherent in this role, and ultimately finds value and meaning in her work.

Julia is a 31-year-old EMD who works for a large paramedical organization in Australia. She has been in her current role for 9 years. She is single and is a Caucasian Australian. As an EMD, Julia is responsible for providing initial response to the caller and dispatching ambulance crews to calls for help that come through the national emergency number. She is a shift worker, which in itself can create challenges to a person's mental and physical health (Stephens & Long, 2000) and although the role is described as "extremely demanding," she loves it; "The job is wonderful, when you get to actually help someone…. It's really cool!" Even though Julia knew what she was getting into when she applied for the job, that knowing was only on paper. The reality of living the job was much, much more than could be accurately imagined. Only a lived experience could really bring the full picture of what it entailed. And only from the experience would she be able to decide if she could do the job well, and if she could withstand the real-life pressures of dealing with multiple, ongoing trauma and crisis from a remote location assisted only by the person she is attempting to help.

THE WORK ROLE

The job is fast paced and high pressured. As an EMD Julia answers one call after the other; the usual caller is in a state of distress and their personal capabilities to attend to the emergency can vary in levels. She must ascertain their emotional and medical status rapidly and accurately so she can use the appropriate tone and questioning. In quick succession she must identify the caller, the location, the problem, and the level of medical severity, often having to create sense out of a chaotic situation over the phone (Adams et al., 2014; Dunford, 2002). EMDs intently use every resource they have available to help. They listen for clues in background sounds and question the caller to allow them to start to visualize and paint a picture of the scene within their own minds. This brings the images of the remote, unseen scenario into their own cognitive realm, creating a visual picture from their remote office. This is done to create avenues or clues so the next steps needed to be provided to the caller can be done with greater accuracy.

Julia will endeavor to enlist her callers as an on-site "tool" or "conduit" to assist her intervention until the paramedics can arrive on the scene. It is an intensive relationship that must be rapidly formed, guided by her voice tone and verbal content. She needs to connect emotionally with the clients, to meet them where they are, and bring them down to a calm, working capacity. This calm has to continue and be monitored so they "don't re-freak," a situation where the caller will calm down and then escalate again once the cognitive reality of the situation loops around in their minds. Keeping control of the caller is of vital importance, necessary to provide her with the most useful asset she has until the paramedics can arrive. Their hands and eyes are for her to use on the scene.

To work in a role that is privy to the fact that death and destruction of lives can occur seemingly by random chance or a "flip of a coin" in life can bring one's own vulnerabilities into stark focus. It can shake their philosophy that the world is generally safe and okay; that health, safety, and vitality are the norm. EMDs have this belief shattered as they become privy to the daily experiences of trauma that occur. They will hear of homicides and abuse as they take place, the last breath of people before they die. EMD's themselves will be abused and accused of killing a patient when the caller needs an outlet for their own trauma. They will have to live the frustration of being unable to coach a traumatized caller to help a dying patient. Other people's traumatic experiences become part of their own lives. The desire to help others in trauma may have been their calling for the role, but the reality is also that they can experience the feelings of loss of control when trying to help others. They are exposed to an ongoing auditory experience of being witness to the real-life tones of pain and grief of others who are in the throes of their own traumatic experiences.

The majority of research conducted with trauma as a focal point and the associated clinical implications or treatment options proposed are done so with an implicit assumption that the experience is either discrete or in the past. For example, prolonged exposure therapy is the most researched intervention for people diagnosed with posttraumatic stress disorder (PTSD; Van Minnen, Harned, Zoellner, & Mills, 2012) and together with other elements of cognitive behavioral therapy is seen as the gold standard for PTSD interventions (Australian Centre for Posttraumatic Mental Health, 2013). However, Julia and others who occupy roles where exposure to potentially traumatic experiences are inherent in the work need to find strategies that maintain their mental health in a context where the threat of trauma and traumatic experiences themselves are a constant. This highlights for clinicians that emergency service professionals and others who work with trauma in an ongoing way need to consider ways to support them with the ongoing nature of trauma in their roles to enable their clients to not only cope with a recent incident of trauma but also respond to future incidences.

Julia expresses an enormous sense of pride for calls that go well; she explains that she often does not gain knowledge of the overall outcome for the patient. When paramedics arrive on the scene the call is terminated. Julia is then left sitting in the office while others at the scene now attend to the emergency. She is immediately expected to move on and take the next incoming call. She reminisced of better times in the past when paramedics would provide EMDs with positive feedback about patient outcomes and how the remote responders involved reacted; "we would do a happy dance!" she laughs with joy at the memories. Also birthing stories where she had to coach those at the scene to deliver a baby that ended well was described as "one of the best moments of my life." Another positive experience was when Julia used her own intuition rather than going with the directed line of questioning (as directed via computer program sequence), which identified the correct cause and helped to save a man's life, "because I asked questions out of sequence and put in 'chest pain', they got to him in time and that was awesome….that was umm, that left me with a glow for days." The positive stories are clearly a part of the job EMDs are initially attracted to when they apply for this role.

Most calls go well but some are harrowing.

TRAUMATIC REACTIONS

Identifying which calls are the most traumatic appears to depend largely on the individual and their own previous experiences and emotional responses to triggers. EMDs cite that they all have their own personal triggers, as seen with Julia's description of hers: "… those teenage suicides, they throw me off my game. They're not the kids with SIDS [sudden infant death syndrome], not the big cases, but the unnecessary ones." Personal connections to a caller's story also reverberated as a traumatic moment. Julia recalled a case that was particularly difficult because she felt an emotional and personal connection to the caller: "There was a call when I first came to [location] who sounded just like my mum and I think that call was a trigger. Like my heart rate went up and when I was off the phone I said I have to get out of here and I think that was what triggered it all." Here Julia is referring to the symptoms of traumatic stress she began to experience. Personal connections can allow for a permeation of their thin but clear professional emotional boundary with the caller. And the caller's trauma can then seep into their own psyche. Unfortunately this was the beginning of a number of events that would increase her symptoms and challenge her mental health.

Compounding elements can increase the exposure to potentially traumatizing experiences in the job, and within a very large emergency service organization it is not unusual to lose a member of your own team. As noted in the opening vignette of this chapter, this also happened to Julia. A colleague who had been battling with a mental health issue but had worn a "mask" in the workplace to hide his distress suddenly committed suicide. Julia was left traumatized by this experience. However, the nature of her work meant that the potential for trauma simply kept coming. She shared that it was not long after losing her colleague that she hit a run of what she perceived to be "horrible, senseless deaths," where her sadness and grief bubbled up to the surface. Julia described her difficulty coping after her colleague's death as experiences of "pure insomnia, it was pure, I didn't sleep and my body would give up after about 5 or 6 days." She describes a succession of provoking calls soon after her colleague's suicide, including a teenager who jumped from a balcony, another young teenager who hung herself, and a baby who was so severely abused that it went into a coma and they turned the machines off. These were further triggers of senseless deaths for her. Despite these triggers occurring, Julia voiced how she could place her feelings aside at the time of the call, because the person on the line becomes the priority "when people are scared they need to know someone is there for them." She describes this as an established cycle of dealing with trauma: "I learned to cope by I shut myself off, but that was my coping mechanisms since I was really young. I would shut myself down and do the job. But being an EMD will push your buttons no matter what issues you have."

Julia's own emotional reactions are described as being put to the side during calls but the trauma is still felt in a delayed manner: "Its only when you're driving home you can let it impact you. And well you can't be crying down on the motorway *(laughter)* because you know, you have to get home." The reaction to trauma can be just below the surface, although where small triggers can set things off: "I hate seeing animals on the side of the road on nights like that. That breaks it. It breaks that crack. Like you see someone's dog or cat. I hate it. I absolutely hate it. I think sometimes I'm soppier about animals than I am about people now, maybe because you can give so much love to your animals, but yeah that gets distressing." Experiences of isolation from others is also a trauma reaction that can be experienced by EMDs, as Julia's own experiences provide example for: "I have to physically push it back [emotional reactions to trauma], push it down, and rather than letting it go later when I'm not at work which I am supposed to do, I basically carry it into my private life and put barriers up and they're permanently up. So I try not to get too close to people. I don't communicate extremely well with other people. My interpersonal relationships, my new ones, are very ah (pause) uninvested, is probably the term I would use." This isolation can form as a protective factor, but it also limits their own potential positive connections with others. The isolation and dissociation that Julia describes is also one of the known negative effects of trauma (e.g., Grant, Beck, MarquesPalyo, & Clapp, 2008).

Given that Julia works in this context, understanding her own responses to trauma is vital. During the interview, Julia provided insights into her level of personal reflection and understanding. "Umm I'm one of those ones unless it's perfect I get anxious *(laughter)* I am in a permanent state of anxiety." She reflects how she understands why she becomes anxious and the physical and psychological symptoms of her distress: "When I don't have enough resources and things don't go perfectly I tend to get very stressed, very anxious and I get insomnia." Julia reflects that she still to this day does not know the call that was the exact source of where her gradual breakdown started, but understanding her triggers and subsequent patterns were important to enabling strategies for her to deal with them. Exploring further into the context of traumatic roles and the personal and organizational responsibilities placed on the individual can uncover more information and context.

ORGANIZATIONAL CONTEXT

Narratives of other EMDs (Adams et al., 2014) have identified that there is a unified belief that the responsibility for each call lies on the EMD's shoulder each time they pick up the phone, not only as a sense of moral and personal responsibility and care, but also because Julia and her colleagues are also constantly monitored—everything they do, say, advise, express, every key stroke is recorded. These monitoring processes can be implemented without warning, creating a perception of a "Big Brother" work environment, as Julia explains: "Well, I came back from holiday and that's when I was officially informed that the watch-desk was watching." Although she voiced her understanding for the need for such scrutiny from accountability and training perspectives, it adds a layer of pressure to an already pressured job. "Big Brother" expects rapid turnarounds for crews and fast response times to calls. When a crew is not available when needed, the EMD is questioned as to what they are doing about the workload.

The operational aspects of the role create enormous amounts of personal and work-related pressure. In addition, there is the potential for litigation and appearances in a Coroner's court where other EMDs have described this experience as being terrifying and isolating, with minimal support provided from the organization, giving a sense of "washed hands" from the organization when a potential flailing may arise (Adams et al., 2014). The EMD narratives of "Big Brother" and elevated vigilance highlight experiences of pressure whereby they are responsible for another person's life on multiple levels. And this continues every day, often repeatedly over a work day for them. This mirrors the pressures currently known and perhaps more clearly understood through research with firefighters, paramedics, and police who also have high levels of responsibilities for life (e.g., Armstrong, Shakespeare-Finch, & Shochet, 2014; Jonsson & Segesten, 2004; Sofianopoulous,

Williams, & Archer, 2010). So this brings forward the question of how EMDs find ways to cope with the long-term and multifaceted stresses of working with people experiencing trauma and how EMDs and other emergency service personnel make sense of the work that they do.

SENSE OF COHERENCE

Emergency workers cannot change the nature of their work role, including exposure to potential trauma, and therefore they need to find ways of dealing with the nature of their work. When the context cannot be changed (e.g., potential trauma, shift work) the promotion and maintenance of a person's mental health necessarily becomes one of managing cognitive, emotional, and behavioral responses to the challenges. Antonovsky (1979) provided a useful framework for thinking about dealing with the ever-present stressors in life, from trauma to pollution and disease, in maintaining health. He suggested that the origins of health, which he called salutogenic factors, are most easily dealt with if a person has, or can develop, a strong sense of coherence (SOC) and that the stronger the coherence or meaning making about the event, the stronger the person's ability is to deal with distress. SOC comprises three overarching components: comprehensibility, manageability, and meaningfulness (Antonovsky, 1979). Comprehension refers to a person's ability to make "sense" of the event. Manageability is the sense that one's internal and external resources are sufficient to meet the demands of the challenges they are confronted with. Meaningfulness refers to the individual's ability to see events as challenges and accept these as worthy of investing energy. The theory suggests that there is a dynamic interplay between these three core components of SOC and that all three domains are needed to be equally balanced for optimal health. For example, health will be compromised if a person can make sense of an event but not manage the experience or bestow a sense of meaning, or if they can bestow meaning and comprehend the event but not manage it.

Using Julia as the case study, there are indications in her interview that suggested she sometimes struggles to comprehend the nature of her work. For example, she recalls teenage suicide as an example that essentially "throw[s] me off my game." It is the senselessness of this loss of life that challenges Julia's mental health. Julia also speaks about how she manages her work and readily admits that some of her ways of managing it are not conducive to mental health. For example, she states she is "in a permanent state of anxiety" and that she has "learned to cope by I shut myself off." However, she is confident in her capacity to execute her role, for example, the story she recounts of overriding the automated questioning system that resulted in saving the life of a patient with chest pain. But it is perhaps the meaningfulness that is the most protective for Julia in guarding her mental health. As the definition of this component suggests, she sees her role as a challenge and that the energy she puts into her role is worth the psychological and physical investment she makes. Julia also keeps the positive aspects of her job in the forefront of her mind. Although she struggles to comprehend the senselessness of some events, she remains mindful of the value of her work. For example, she recalled finding out that a job had gone well and was "doing a happy dance" as well as the joy of some calls such as coaching a caller to successfully deliver a baby.

However, taken together, it appears that Julia does not have all of the components of this model in equal balance. Although she successfully creates meaning around her role and the experiences it has given her, the challenge orientation she adopts, and the reliance on peers and supervisors to manage the role, she still struggles to comprehend some of the trauma she bears witness to and admits that her strategies for coping are not always successful. Julia admits to having chronic insomnia at times and to living in a state of heightened arousal. Her admission to shying away from developing intimate relationships as a way of protecting herself also raises questions about her overall well-being. What is also useful about taking a salutogenic approach to understanding health is that negative influences and sometimes lasting detrimental outcomes of exposure to stress and trauma do not negate the potential for the same experiences to be a catalyst for positive personal changes. Indeed positive posttrauma changes, termed posttraumatic growth (Calhoun & Tedeschi, 2013; Tedeschi & Calhoun, 1995), are a more common outcome of emergency service work than pathology like PTSD (Shakespeare-Finch, Smith, Gow, Embelton, & Baird, 2003).

POSTTRAUMATIC GROWTH

According to Calhoun and Tedeschi's model of posttraumatic growth (2013) the capacity to accept a situation as transpired, engaging in effortful rumination, receiving support, and bestowing the experience with meaning are vital components in promoting growth. EMDs explore finding their own ways to acceptance of the trauma they witness daily and reframe their work role so they can, to an efficient extent, explain the unexplainable—why some people are suddenly involved in senseless death. The acceptance extends to accepting the limits of their role, events, and their own vulnerability. This has been described as essentially a unique and personal journey for them (Adams et al., 2014). As Julia and others have expressed, the first 1–2 years on the job is when the impacts of the job role and trauma really first hit them. And following this is their own reframing and making sense of all they witness and experience, which often occurs in a relatively simple and succinct form. As described by Julia "I'm just learning to relax that a bit and be realistic in my expectations of myself and others. And to learn that things are never perfect no matter how hard you try they are not perfect."

Acceptance of her own vulnerability as a human being who experiences emotions and has her own reactions because of her own experiences was another significant element. Julia clearly understands the types of calls that have a traumatic impact on her and that an apparently personal connection gives rise to significant difficulty as was the case when the caller sounded like her mother. With time Julia and others in her role understand that having a call that triggers their own emotional reactions does not mean that they are not good at their job. Living a full and whole life themselves means that sometimes issues in their life will mirror that of the caller. Be it a death, a birth, a tone, or similar situation, any personal connection with the story has the ability to trigger their own emotional trauma. EMDs who protect themselves by shutting themselves down in their personal lives and become cold and uncaring are potentially at greater risk of ongoing trauma.

ORGANIZATIONAL SUPPORT

The employing organization has an important role in monitoring the mental health of their staff and in providing appropriate support to successfully negotiate the trauma personnel face. Looking to the salutogenic framework and SOC, manageability of the trauma requires accessibility to their own internal and external resources. With Julia's story this was initiated through the use of self-reflections. This inner awareness and observations of her own reactions, emotions, and behaviors related to health and well-being enabled her to identify a need for external resources to assist in managing and coping with the trauma she had experienced. Julia describes how her self-reflections enabled her to seek out support and the range of ways she gains support: "I talk to my dogs. And some friends. And I've been talking to a psychologist [provided by the organization]. And that's why [after her colleague died] I went and saw her because I knew the cycle and when that occurs I get insomnia and I'm up for days. I needed some help with that. To try and figure out once and for all where it was coming from and how to put coping strategies in place so I can have a wonderful full life and know what to do when that happens."

Talking to a professional for support was not described as always being easy. Julia describes her sessions as "Stressful!" then laughs and continues "No she's [psychologist] wonderful but she pushes those buttons and makes me work for it *(laughter)* it's probably one of the best things about this organisation that I appreciate, to have that back-up." Emergency workers will often seek assistance from external supports outside of the work place, including friends, colleagues, and family members, but only if they have a similar background that they believe enables the support person to be able to withstand their own "normal" work day (e.g., counselor, nurse, paramedic). Understanding that an emergency worker's role is not "normal" and the need to protect others is often a barrier to using partners also for support (Adams et al., 2014). Julia explains this as: "Because no matter how close you are to your partner you just can't. Generally it's horrific and they just don't get it."

ADDITIONAL COPING STRATEGIES

Manageability of trauma through a range of internal and external resources and support systems to assist Julia to form coping skills is a necessary part of the SOC framework for health and well-being. A strategy used by many people who work in this type of occupation is humor, most notably, the use of "black humor." This is described as being inappropriate, crass, and maybe even somewhat crude, but ultimately necessary to help emergency workers to break free of a fixation on the senselessness of an unexplained traumatic event they witness, especially for hard-to-comprehend cases, those that really could cause ongoing trauma for the worker. It is also sometimes just to break the intensity of the moment or relentless exposure of traumas. This is a "behind closed doors" coping mechanism, understood only by those who experience the role. It is a careful guarded coping mechanism as it is never meant for public ears because of the potential to misunderstand the basis and use of humor and potentially offend. Julia articulates this as: "Excessive humour really helps. It's really, really important. If I didn't have that sense of humour I would go absolutely batty. It's the only way to vent [between each other] without being offensive to anyone." The need to put in place supports and coping mechanisms is perceived to be vital to mental health as there is an understanding Julia voices that anyone in this role can be at risk of having a psychological breakdown if they bottle up their emotional reactions to the trauma they are exposed to.

Julia verbalized this through a deep desire "to figure out where it all comes from [her reactions to some traumas and not others]," so she can make sense of the trauma and have her own coping mechanisms in place that will support her to have what she desires for "a wonderful life," to be a fully functioning person with positive health and well-being. So when those "buttons" that come along with the role are pushed, she can make sense and place meaning upon them.

Julia's story so far lists the first two components of the SOC, making sense of the event and using internal and external coping skills. But how does she create meaning out of random chaos? Although acceptance of traumatic events allows EMDs to comprehend the reality of what they experience, making meaning of these experiences through effortful rumination or forming new narratives holds the potential for long-term health and well-being to be able to work in this role. New narratives are a vital part of growth (Calhoun & Tedeschi, 2013; Tedeschi & Calhoun, 1995). Even when outcomes are not positive for the patient, EMDs have described how they use self-talk and self-reflection to form new narratives to help them understand a senseless death or situation that they could not control through a reframing of the initial situation to find value in what they provided (Adams et al., 2014). This can be from effortful rumination after a call, conducted over a short or long time frame. When there is a negative outcome for the patient, EMDs have discussed how they find their own sense of meaning. This can include considering how their efforts ensured some small positive, like finding out that a successful organ donation was possible to assist another patient or reflecting that they enabled the patient to live just long enough for the family to say good-bye. No matter how small it is, they hold onto this philosophy that they have made a difference in someone's life. And to do this many have to let go of their desire and initial beliefs that they could have absolute control over the outcome by providing the right instructions to the caller; that they could save them.

SOME OF JULIA'S GROWTH

Consistent with the model of posttraumatic growth (Calhoun & Tedeschi, 2013) EMDs and other emergency service workers describe an increased appreciation of life by enjoying time with those they love and care for after their previous beliefs about life longevity, safety, and health are shattered (e.g., Armstrong et al., 2014; Regehr, Goldberg, & Hughes, 2002; Shakespeare-Finch, 2012). These relationships can be described as now being of a quality and attentiveness that they had not experienced or felt before taking this role, whether with family, friends, or others. Although Julia currently struggles to form new friendships from a protective wall she has placed around herself, her voice is filled with love when she discusses her connection with her pets after work "I hang with my dogs, seriously they are both caring and active and they are happy stupid." Her appreciation for the long-term close friends and family whom she can rely on and talk to has a genuine richness to it—a valued external resource she can cherish. This new appreciation of life links to self-care, allowing the time, resources, and permission needed to look after themselves, both physically and psychologically.

For a clinician, supporting clients like Julia to find their own sense of meaning can be pivotal to their current and future associations with trauma. This can be achieved by facilitating the formation of new cognitive strategies of acceptance and meaning making that are unique to their own interests and supported by their own individual coping skills (Calhoun & Tedeschi, 2013). These elements may be paramount to Julia on her journey toward well-being. As Julia reflects her own changes with the help of psychological support "I'm just learning to relax that a bit and be realistic in my expectations of myself and to learn that things are never perfect no matter how hard you try." Understanding herself and her desire to control outcomes is significant in these first steps toward psychological health: "I like things to be black and white, and our job is grey." For Julia, this is where she struggles and can find herself stuck, with her difficulty to embrace the acceptance that she cannot control the outcome. This goes against her previously formed beliefs that if she just makes the right choice of black or white, she can achieve the desired consequence. This belief no longer holds fast, and so she begins her journey to find a new philosophy.

Learning to cope when things do not go the way she wants, and embracing the "gray" of life in other activities can now be seen in Julia's uptake of a new hobby: "I attempt to garden, it doesn't work, they die *(laughter)*. I tend to care too much for my plants *(laughter)*. My healthy ones are my attempts to garden." Challenging her desire to have complete control over her garden so that all of her plants would live as an after work activity, using both humor and allowing the beginning of acceptance in the fact she cannot save all of her plants, literally and metaphorically reflects Julia's attempt to create new meaning around her work. The activity acts to validate the knowledge that she deeply and sincerely wants to save them all. Here, Julia shows her personal characteristic of a positive sense of humor as a way of transforming this ability to accept life and death into her world at both home and work. Alterations to self-perception, strengthening, and forming new philosophies of life that are concurrent with her current life experiences in her work role can be important steps toward growth rather than ongoing or retriggering traumatic symptoms. And this may be the important stepping stone she needs before finding her own sense of meaning.

SUMMARY

To demonstrate meaning and posttraumatic growth in this chapter it would have been easier to have used an interview with an EMD, paramedic, or other emergency service person who was full of signs of growth and meaning making. Instead we chose Julia because her interview more accurately reflects the complexities of maintaining and promoting psychological well-being when working in an environment that constantly challenges the worker's mental health. Importantly, growth is not an either/or outcome of exposure to trauma. Ongoing distress, the creation of new narratives, the gaining of wisdom, engaging in effortful rumination, and using strategies and resources that help to negotiate life where the potential for trauma is inherent in the work role is an ongoing process. Julia clearly has struggled and to some extent continues to do so. It is through that struggle that meaning is created and positive personal changes are made.

REFERENCES

Adams, K., Shakespeare-Finch, J., & Armstrong, D. (2014). An interpretative phenomenological analysis of stress and well-being in emergency medical dispatchers. *Journal of Loss and Trauma*. http://dx.doi.org/10.1080/15325024.2014.949141 (advanced online view).

Antonovsky, A. (1979). *Health, stress and coping: New perspectives on mental and physical well-being*. San Francisco: Jossey-Bass.

Armstrong, D., Shakespeare-Finch, J., & Shochet, I. (2014). Predicting posttraumatic growth and posttraumatic stress in fire-fighters. *Australian Journal of Psychology, 66*, 38–46. http://dx.doi.org/10.1111/ajpy.12032.

Australian Centre for Posttraumatic Mental Health. (2013). *The Australian guidelines for the treatment of acute stress disorder and posttraumatic stress disorder*. http://phoenixaustralia.org/wp-content/uploads/2015/03/ACPMH-Guidelines.pdf.

Calhoun, L., & Tedeschi, R. (2013). *Posttraumatic growth in clinical practice*. New York: Routledge.

Dunford, J.V. (2002). Emergency medical dispatch. *Emergency Medicine Clinics of North America, 20*, 859–875. http://dx.doi.org/10.1016/S0733-8627(02)00032-9.

Grant, D. M., Beck, J. G., Marques, L., Palyo, S. A., & Clapp, J. D. (2008). The structure of distress following trauma: posttraumatic stress disorder, major depressive disorder, and generalized anxiety disorder. *Journal of Abnormal Psychology, 117,* 662–672. http://dx.doi.org/10.1037/a0012591.

Jonsson, A., & Segesten, K. (2004). Daily stress and concept of self in Swedish ambulance personnel. *Prehospital and Disaster Medicine, 19,* 226–234. http://dx.doi.org/10.1017/S1049023X00001825.

Regehr, C., Goldberg, G., & Hughes, J. (2002). Exposure to human tragedy, empathy, and trauma in ambulance paramedics. *American Journal of Orthopsychiatry, 72,* 505–513. http://dx.doi.org/10.1037/0002-9432.72.4.505.

Shakespeare-Finch, J. (2012). First responders and trauma. In C. Figley (Ed.), *The encyclopaedia of trauma.* London, UK: Sage.

Shakespeare-Finch, J., Rees, A., & Armstrong, D. (2014). Social support, self-efficacy, trauma and well-being in emergency medical dispatchers. *Social Indicators Research.* http://dx.doi.org/10.1007/s11205-014-0749-9.

Shakespeare-Finch, J. E., Smith, S. G., Gow, K. M., Embelton, G., & Baird, L. (2003). The prevalence of posttraumatic growth in emergency ambulance personnel. *Traumatology, 9,* 58–70.

Sofianopoulos, S., Williams, B., & Archer, F. (2010). Paramedics and the effects of shift work on sleep: a literature review. *Emergency Medicine Journal, 29,* 152–155. http://dx.doi.org/10.1136/emj.2010.094342.

Stephens, C., & Long, N. (2000). Communication with police supervisors and peers as a buffer of work-related traumatic stress. *Journal of Organizational Behavior, 21,* 407–424. http://dx.doi.org/10.1002/(SICI)1099-1379(200006)21:4<407::AID-JOB17>3.0.CO;2-N.

Tedeschi, R. G., & Calhoun, L. G. (1995). *Trauma and transformation: Growing in the aftermath of suffering.* California: SAGE.

Van Minnen, A., Harned, M., Zoellner, l., & Mills, K. (2012). Examining potential contraindications for prolonged exposure therapy for PTSD. *European Journal of Psychotraumatology, 3.* http://dx.doi.org/10.3402/ejpt.v3i0.18805 (advanced online view).

CHAPTER 9

Meaning Making Concerning Acquired Disability

B.A. Tallman[1,2], A.C. Hoffman[3,4]

[1]Coe College, Cedar Rapids, IA, United States; [2]UnityPoint Health-St. Luke's Hospital, Cedar Rapids, United States; [3]University of Iowa, Iowa City, IA, United States; [4]University of Illinois at Urbana-Champaign, Champaign, IL, United States

Shirley is an African American female in her mid-30s who recently moved to a small Midwestern community to get away from the violence and gang activity prevalent in her neighborhood in a large metropolitan area. She has two adolescent children, and she wanted to raise them in a stable living environment with excellent education and access to good health care. As a single mother, she works 12-h days at a factory to financially support her family. During the day, her aunt provides child care, but beyond her aunt, her support network is limited. She has limited contact with her family, as they live several hours away in a large Midwestern city. Being a minority in a predominately Caucasian area, she frequently feels out of place. In the past, she has experienced clinical depression, and she has a history of using alcohol to cope with psychosocial stressors.

One morning, on her way to work on a two-lane road, a truck passed the center lane and struck her small two-door sedan head-on. The car was completely destroyed, but miraculously, Shirley survived. She does not remember the accident itself, partially due to the traumatic brain injury (TBI) she sustained. Following the accident, her thinking was "fuzzy" due to posttraumatic amnesia (PTA), and she could not fully comprehend or grasp the severity of her situation. Shirley was diagnosed with a new T6 complete spinal cord injury (SCI) resulting in paraplegia.

Her first several weeks were spent at a regional trauma center to medically stabilize her. As her cognition began to clear, she understood her deficits and her depression worsened. She was transferred to an acute rehabilitation unit where she began the long road to recovery and to live independently. At times, she perceived that the staff treated her differently because of her ethnicity and background. She felt like she no longer had control of anything in her

Reconstructing Meaning After Trauma
ISBN 978-0-12-803015-8
http://dx.doi.org/10.1016/B978-0-12-803015-8.00009-7

133

life, including her bowel and bladder functioning. Her future was plagued with uncertainty. She struggled to make sense of the aftermath of her situation. Multiple questions and intrusive thoughts attacked her on a daily basis. Will I ever walk again? How will I care for my family? How will I live my life from a wheelchair? How do I make sense of all of this?

As Shirley progressed through her rehabilitation, she began to construct meaning, to create goals and a new life story. She made the decision to be "better off after my injury than before." She made it her mission to work as hard as she could so she would walk out of the hospital. Shirley's narrative turned from despair that her life was over, to hope for the future. She began to rely heavily on her faith, and she reconnected with individuals via social media to form prayer groups. She prayed on a daily basis. She demonstrated a fighting spirit that she never knew she had; she fought to survive each day. The thought of not being better off than she was before was too demoralizing. Her mission in life became to care for her children; she was going to be the best mother possible. To some, her views of walking again and "being better off than before" were unrealistically optimistic. But for Shirley, less than anything else was not surviving. Her new life narrative focused on serving God, "living life," and being the best parent I can be.

Shirley's story is not unlike many other individuals who have experienced a traumatic event or debilitating chronic illness resulting in an acquired disability. Approximately 56.7 million people had a documented disability in 2010, and of this number, approximately 12.6% or 38.3 million people had a severe disability (Brault, 2012). Approximately 14.9 million people aged 15 years and older have experienced difficulty with seeing, hearing, or speaking (Brault, 2012). Many of these disabilities were acquired and resulted from traumatic injuries or other debilitating medical conditions.

According to the Americans with Disabilities Act (ADA, 1990), a "disability" is defined as a physical or mental impairment that substantially limits one or more of the major life activities of such individual (ADA, Section 1630.2). Individuals with disabilities experience a major disruption in functioning, including completing activities of daily living, such as caring for oneself, seeing, hearing, and eating. Physical disabilities are inclusive of a variety of disorders. For example, someone who has experienced a motorcycle accident, resulting in a lower limb amputation, may not be able to ambulate effectively and suffer from phantom limb pain.

With all the attention given to negative adjustment for individuals with physical disabilities, it is only recently that the influence of the positive psychology movement (e.g., Seligman & Csikszentmihalyi, 2000) has been used to examine individuals with acquired disabilities. The positive psychology movement shifted the focus of posttrauma adaptation from maladaptive adjustment, or emphasizing psychopathology stemming from disability, to positive aspects of human functioning, including resilience, meaning making, benefit finding, and posttraumatic growth.

In addition, although there is ample evidence to indicate that individuals experience negative consequences related to their disability, research suggests that a large proportion of individuals return to a normal baseline level following adverse life events (Bonanno, Westphal, & Mancini, 2011). This return to baseline illustrates how "resilient" individuals can be. Therefore, resilience can be considered achieving stability or returning to one's baseline level of functioning following a traumatic event (Bonanno, 2004). Persons with a SCI could be considered resilient if they initially experience a depressive reaction, but later returned to normal emotional functioning. Although resilience is an important part of psychological functioning, it will not be the focus of this chapter.

Influential researchers and clinicians within the field of rehabilitation psychology have long noted that not all individuals experience deleterious consequences as a result of their disability (Dembo, Leviton, & Wright, 1956; Wright, 1983). There have been many terms to describe an individual experiencing positive change from adversity, or the experience of growth above and beyond a place of resilience. Tedeschi and Calhoun (2004, 2009) coined the term *posttraumatic growth* (PTG) to denote the experience of positive psychological change resulting from traumatic life events. Wright noted that individuals can learn to find acceptance and appreciation in their disability (Wright, 1989). Research suggests that between 30 and 70% of individuals experience at least some positive change in their lives as a result of living through trauma (Weiss & Berger, 2010).

There are several specific domains of PTG. Individuals can experience changes in life perspective or life philosophies. For example, "the little things become more important" is a fairly common response. Individuals frequently note becoming closer with family or friends and experiencing increased closeness in interpersonal relationships. Individuals often describe becoming "stronger" than they thought they were in the domain of personal strength. Experiencing a change in one's spiritual/religious beliefs is also common following growth. Individuals have also experienced changes regarding their health and health behaviors.

This chapter will address the following goals. First, we will provide a brief review of the historical account of growth from a disability or rehabilitation psychology perspective. Although we will review research evidence, our chapter will emphasize clinical and practical interventions practitioners can use with their patients, especially in the early stages of disability. The second primary purpose of the chapter is to briefly review the literature regarding PTG among acquired disability populations. Last, we will provide specific recommendations for clinicians and health care workers who work closely with individuals with acquired disabilities.

GROWTH MODELS IN ACQUIRED DISABILITY

In the past twenty years emphasis has been placed on how the positive psychology movement may impact adjustment to disability and psychological well-being. Several authors and clinicians in the field of rehabilitation psychology have written about positive psychology in the context of adjustment to disability (e.g., Dunn & Dougherty, 2005; Dunn, Uswatte, Elliott, Lastres, & Beard, 2013; Ehde, 2010; Elliott, Kurylo, & Rivera, 2002; Wehmeyer, 2013), with the areas of resiliency, positive emotions (Fredrickson, 2001), and finding growth or meaning from trauma receiving the most attention (Tedeschi & Calhoun, 2004). To cover all facets within positive psychology and disability is well beyond the scope of this chapter, but we will cover finding growth or PTG from acquired disability.

With the practicing clinician in mind, we will review several theories of growth that will conceptualize growth comprehensively, from both "process" and "outcome" perspectives. Tedeschi and Calhoun (1996, 2004, 2009) acknowledge that PTG can follow several trajectories, including one that involves coping. Evidence of different trajectories for growth is supported by discrepancies in the literature regarding growth variables related to positive or negative adjustment: for example, the relationship between growth and adjustment may be moderated by time since trauma or diagnosis (Helgeson, Reynolds, & Tomich, 2006). The process versus outcome distinction of growth is especially important for clinicians who work with individuals in the early stages following traumatic events.

The Janus–Face model conceptualizes growth as having two sides, a constructive side and an illusory side (Zoellner & Maercker, 2006). The constructive side is functional or self-transcending, consistent with Tedeschi and Calhoun's conceptualization of growth. The illusory side may represent self-deception or dysfunction. For example, a man who experienced a TBI may state he wished the injury never happened to him, but because he was injured, he is going to "make the most" of his life and "live each day to its fullest." Research has supported the illusory component of growth among medical populations (e.g., cancer; Widows, Jacobsen, Booth-Jones, & Fields, 2005), with growth being related to defensive denial and avoidance.

Researchers and clinicians have assessed the temporal component of growth, which may aid in distinguishing the process versus outcome nature of this construct (Tallman, 2013; Tallman et al., 2014). Growth at early time points following trauma may represent a positive illusion, or a coping process. Among individuals with SCIs, research suggests that tendencies to deny negative information have been related to less distress, less hostility, and fewer problems associated with disability (Elliot & Richards, 1999). The illusory process may be adaptive in the short term, but if this process continues over time and deliberate attempts are made to avoid reality, then maladjustment may occur (Zoellner & Maercker, 2006). The constructive side, which takes longer to experience, is hypothesized to be linked to positive adjustment. From a cognitive processing perspective, if the illusory process is co-occurring with the constructive side, or if there are conscious attempts to process and make sense of the experience, then the illusory component could be considered sell-palliative and functional.

In the context of the early stages of adjustment to disability, the illusory process may be important for dealing with the initial shock of trauma, particularly in a rehabilitation setting where the focus is often on functional gains. For example, a woman with an acquired brain injury (ABI) who loses her husband in a traumatic motorcycle accident may experience an acute stress reaction along with cognitive deficits. She may also begin to believe that this catastrophic event will help her regain control in her life, and that she has to continue moving forward. In addition, she may become more present with her family and friends and promise to spend more time with loved ones. If attempts at coping are successful, then the constructive component of growth should increase over time, whereas illusory components decrease, leading to positive adjustment and increased personal well-being (Zoellner & Maercker, 2006).

Individuals with disabilities may experience PTG and a sense of purpose in their lives, with new levels of functioning (postdisability) surpassing pre-event levels of functioning. In her seminal book titled *Physical Disability: A Psychological Approach,* Beatrice Wright laid the groundwork for rehabilitation psychology. Wright's (1983) theory focused on understanding disability as an interaction between the person and the social context. Wright's work has influenced the articulation of personal growth and positive adaptation from disability (Elliott, Kurylo, & Riveria, 2002). Specifically, individuals can experience new meaning and value in their lives through acceptance

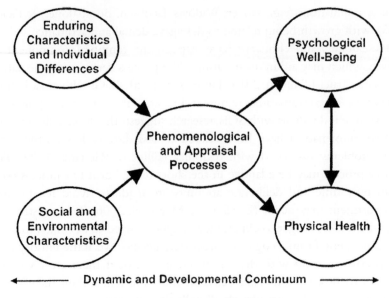

Figure 9.1 Dynamic model of growth.

and appreciation of their disability (Wright, 1989). Consistent with Tedeschi and Calhoun's model (2004), Wright's view of value changes and self-understanding in response to disability represents similar domains that have been empirically investigated using both quantitative (e.g., Posttraumatic Growth Inventory; Tedeschi & Calhoun, 1996) and qualitative methods (e.g., Hefferon, Grealy, & Mutrie, 2009).

Elliott et al. (2002) developed an integrative dynamic model to more fully conceptualize positive growth and adjustment from a rehabilitation psychology perspective (see Fig. 9.1). A central tenant to their model emphasizes the person and environment relationship (e.g., Wright, 1983), including how psychosocial variables (e.g., demographic, behavioral patterns) impact adaptation from disability and experiencing growth or meaning. Their model conceptualizes disability in several broad-based domains—enduring characteristics and individual differences; social and environmental characteristics; phenomenological and appraisal processes; psychological well-being; and physical health—with each domain dynamically interacting with one another.

The first domain, enduring characteristics and individual differences, addresses demographic characteristics, disability-related characteristics (e.g., pain concerns), predisability behavioral patterns, and personality characteristics. An example of a predisability behavioral pattern is someone with a history of using drugs or alcohol who may abuse substances to deal with the disability. Regarding demographic variables, younger age and more recent disability have been associated with greater risk of depression in people with disabilities (Bombardier et al., 2010). Variables such as hope (Snyder, 1989), defensive denial (Elliott & Richards, 1999), positive illusions (Elliott & Richards, 1999; Tallman et al., 2013), and more traditional personality characteristics are also included in the model (e.g., neuroticism and extraversion; Krause & Rohe, 1998).

The second domain, social and interpersonal environment, encompasses factors such as social support, environmental barriers, and social stereotypes. Social support has received a considerable amount of attention within the broader literature related to health outcomes, and more specifically in the context of disability populations. A review of the literature among chronic illness populations—diabetes, asthma, heart disease, and epilepsy—revealed a modest positive relationship between social support and chronic illness self-management (Gallant, 2003). Among individuals treated for heart failure, research suggests that decreased levels of socials support are linked to hospital readmission and mortality (Luttik et al., 2005).

Social/environmental characteristics are believed to have a considerable influence on the phenomenological and appraisal processes, the third domain. The phenomenological and appraisal processes domain focuses on the perception and appraisal of stress in the model, and is germane in the process of growth. The appraisal of stress has long been a hallmark feature of stress and coping theory (e.g., Lazarus & Folkman, 1984), and within the current model appraisal is believed to have considerable influence on adjustment to disability. The current model purports that the processes of achieving growth become first evident when individuals evaluate and begin making sense of their situation (Elliott et al., 2002). The authors speculate this coping process is at the core of individuals beginning to make sense of their situation, turning inward to regain control, and seeking growth from their disability (Kennedy et al., 2000).

The final two domains of the model are related to adjustment following disability, and share considerable overlap: psychological well-being and physical health. Psychological well-being has historically taken into account measures of distress, including anxiety and depression, psychosocial impairment, and marital discord or divorce. Overall, physical health is purported to contribute to more positive outcomes such as self-esteem, acceptance of disability, and life satisfaction.

Qualitative research methods have examined growth and meaning from acquired disability. Salick and Auerbach (2006) conducted semistructured interviews with individuals diagnosed with multiple sclerosis, below-knee amputations, visual impairment, and SCIs and identified five theoretical constructs of recovery. The authors posit that visibly disabled individuals progress through various phases or "stages" from the initial trauma toward recovery. The first stage, apprehension, is the sense that something is wrong. This stage encompasses the emotional reaction of not knowing what is wrong with the body to not fully registering the extent of their situation or disability. Feeling the full impact of the diagnosis and its devastation is the second stage, and this is the stage in which individuals experience the failure of their body and loss of physical self. The third stage, choosing to go on, captures the individuals' existential presence to move on in life. This stage is characterized by individuals finding their inner strength and creating plans of action to move forward in life. The fourth stage, building a way to live, includes coping mechanisms to carry out decisions in their lives and address themes of creating a support system, using humor, and locating hope. It is within this stage that the authors theorize that individuals experience personal meaning from their disability, which in turn allows them to begin making sense and take control of their situation. The last stage, integration of the trauma and expansion of the self, examines themes of acceptance and moving forward with their disability. The authors purport that additional themes of growth emerge in this stage, including wanting to contribute and give something back to community, enhancement of personal empathy from one's own experience, and a general sense of increased purpose and meaning in life.

As one participant stated:

I feel like I'm a better person. I like myself better now. I just feel like, as horrible as it is, and I wouldn't wish it upon anyone, suffering does make you grow. It gives you a certain depth and maturity and adds another element to your personality that wasn't there before. You become more creative, deeper. You just access other parts of yourself so that your self is bigger than it was before. (pg. 1033–1034)

ACQUIRED DISABILITY AND GROWTH

The following section reviews the PTG literature across several types of acquired disability: visual impairment, SCI, TBI, amputation, burn injuries, pain conditions, and cardiac events. Factors related and leading to growth are presented to help clinicians maximize opportunities for positive adjustment to disability.

Visual Impairment

Few studies have examined positive change after visual impairment. One study of changes following visual impairment found that negative changes were reported three times more often than positive changes in a variety of life domains (Boerner, Wang, & Cimarolli, 2006). Positive changes included increased compassion and empathy for others, increased self-worth, greater appreciation of life, and placing higher priority on family. Age may also play a factor in growth following vision loss. Boerner and Wang (2010) found that middle-aged adults reported experiencing more changes, both positive and negative, compared with older-aged adults following visual impairment.

Spinal Cord Injury

A landmark longitudinal study indicated those with SCI experience growth, particularly in the realm of personal strength (Pollard & Kennedy, 2007), but total mean levels of self-reported growth were significantly lower compared with breast cancer survivors (Cordova, Cunningham, Carlson, & Andrykowski, 2001). The authors hypothesized that growth may be more difficult to achieve from ongoing traumatic situations compared with traumatic situations that occurred in the past. The study also reported that mental disengagement, depression, and active coping accounted for 48% of the variance in growth, consistent with previous research identifying post-traumatic stress and various coping strategies as correlates of growth. Leisure activities may also play a role in the experience of growth after SCI. One study indicated leisure activities provide opportunities to discover personal strengths, develop meaningful relationships, make sense of trauma and find meaning in everyday life, and generate positive emotions (Chun & Lee, 2010).

Traumatic Brain Injury

Growth has been examined in people with TBI and those who have experienced a stroke. Gangstad, Norman, and Barton (2009) found that growth was positively associated with the coping styles of positive cognitive restructuring, downward comparison, resolution, and denial. They also reported that as time since stroke increased, the relationship between growth and downward comparisons and resolutions became more positive and significant. The study of growth after TBI and ABI has also garnered research interest. Silva et al. (2011) reported that greater levels of subjective impairment at discharge following ABI predicted PTG at 6 months postdischarge. Another longitudinal study among individuals with TBI found that social support, shifts toward spiritual values, new and stable relationships, and activities such as work were correlates of PTG (Powell, Gilson, & Collin, 2012). Finally, PTG after ABI has also been associated with adaptive coping strategies, lower levels of distress, and stronger beliefs about the controllability of brain injury aftereffects through treatment (Rogan, Fortune, & Prentice, 2013).

Amputation

Recent research indicates growth after amputation (e.g., Dunn, 1996; Oaksford et al., 2005). Phelps, Williams, Raichle, Turner, and Ehde (2008) conducted a longitudinal study that found positive cognitive processing reported within 9 weeks of amputation significantly predicted growth at 12 months. The relationship between growth and amputation has also been examined among veterans. Benetato (2011) reported that rumination and perceived social support postdeployment were correlated with PTG among veterans who experienced amputation. In addition, Tuncay and Musabak (2015) found that problem-focused coping was positively associated with all PTG areas, whereas emotion-focused coping was negatively associated with positive changes to relationships with others, among Turkish military veterans with lower limb amputation. In summary, although time since amputation does not seem to be related to growth, certain coping strategies are significant correlates.

Burn Injuries

Rosenbach and Renneberg (2008) examined PTG among people who had been treated for severe burn injury. Participants reported moderate levels of perceived growth, with women reporting significantly higher levels of growth than men. Consistent with previous research, the strongest correlate with growth was active coping and social support. In an examination of growth postburn, Baillie, Sellwood, and Wisely (2014) found location of the burn had a significant effect on growth; those who reported burns on both their hands and face reported significantly higher growth compared with participants who experienced burns on their body or on their face alone. Active coping, perceived social support, and, contrary to previous findings, avoidance coping were identified as significant predictors of growth. The authors suggested avoidance coping may be an appropriate method to deal with pain or scarring from a burn, or perhaps it was associated with posttraumatic stress, which was positively correlated with growth.

Pain Conditions

PTG has been examined in several chronic pain populations, including individuals with fibromyalgia and rheumatoid arthritis (RA). The literature suggests one common form of growth among individuals with RA is the perception of interpersonal benefits. In a longitudinal study of the positive effects of RA on interpersonal relationships, interpersonal benefit finding was associated with less pain, lower psychological distress, and fewer social constraints (Danoff-Burg & Revenson, 2005). Qualitative studies have revealed themes of personal growth after living with fibromyalgia. One study of Swedish women with fibromyalgia or chronic fatigue syndrome found half of the sample described positive aspects of their illness experiences, including increased empathy for the ill, increased self-respect and integrity, and an enhanced sense of what is important in life (Asbring, 2001).

Cardiac Events

Growth has also been reported among those who have experienced cardiac events (e.g., myocardial infarction, coronary artery disease). A prospective study of 1497 Canadian outpatients with coronary artery disease (CAD) reported that being an ethnocultural minority, being younger, lower family income, lower functional status, and fewer depressive symptoms were significantly related to increased levels of PTG (Leung, Gravely-Witte, Macpherson, Irvine, Stewart, & Grace, 2010). Interestingly, growth was also significantly associated with the perception that treatment could control cardiac illness and that CAD symptoms are less cyclical and related to greater consequences. Similarly, Garnefski et al. (2008) found growth was negatively associated with depressive symptoms and positively associated with well-being, extraversion, conscientiousness, and lower neuroticism, as well as the coping strategies positive refocusing, positive reappraisal, and putting into perspective.

INTERVENTIONS TO FACILITATE GROWTH AND RECOMMENDATIONS FOR CLINICIANS

Some evidence suggests psychosocial interventions may nurture PTG (Roepke, 2015). Tedeschi and McNally (2011) presented a theoretical intervention to directly facilitate growth among combat veterans. The intervention model comprises five elements: (1) understanding the trauma response as a precursor to growth, (2) emotional regulation interventions,

(3) constructive self-disclosure, (4) developing a trauma narrative that includes PTG domains, and (5) developing resilient ways of thinking and life principles. Calhoun and Tedeschi (2012) have suggested integrating narrative/constructive and existential approaches into cognitive-behavioral trauma treatments to go beyond reducing symptoms to facilitate PTG. They urged clinicians to take on the role of expert companion in therapy, or "companions who offer some expertise in nurturing naturally occurring processes of healing and growth" (Calhoun & Tedeschi, 2012, p. 23). Expert companions listen to the trauma narrative without trying to solve it, listen for themes of growth and help the client articulate growth if it is present, inquire about the possibility of growth when appropriate, and choose words when discussing growth that reflect that growth comes from the struggle to cope with trauma, not from the trauma itself. Although theoretical in nature, these suggestions paint a clearer picture of how growth may be directly nurtured in a therapeutic environment.

As mentioned, we believe one of the key ways to help facilitate growth is by being an "expert companion" (Calhoun & Tedeschi, 2012) by helping individuals construct a new life narrative following their disability. Clinicians can play a key role in helping individuals craft this new life narrative, especially in the early stages following a traumatic medical event or life-changing medical diagnosis. The following section will focus on specific recommendations for clinicians to work with their clients or patients in the immediate aftermath of the acquired disability. Elliott and colleagues' (2002) model will be used as a framework for clinicians to work from in the context of the rehabilitation environment, or in the immediate aftermath of acquiring a disability.

Individuals may be in disbelief, disarray, and have a very difficult time comprehending the gravity of their situation in the immediate aftermath following an acquired disability. Acute medical problems need to be resolved and the individual needs to be medically stable before the long and sometimes arduous rehabilitation process. In this immediate stage it is important for clinicians to begin to assess the patient's level of understanding of their disability or their underlying illness. Referring back to Shirley, in the early stages of responding to a spinal cord and traumatic brain injury, there is a tremendous amount of information to comprehend (e.g., nutrition, bowel/bladder management, skin care) while recovering from medical issues (e.g., posttraumatic amnesia) and adjusting to psychosocial stressors (e.g., financial concerns due to inability to work). Consistent with the enduring characteristics and individual differences domain (Elliot et al., 2002), assessing the extent to which Shirley comprehends information may help the clinician gauge her individual response to disability, and how her preexisting assumptions about life and future goals have been challenged (Tedeshi & Calhoun, 2004). Having an understanding of Shirley's personality characteristics (e.g., internal versus external locus of control), behavioral patterns, and life assumptions may help the clinician determine how well she is integrating this new information into their reality.

In the social and interpersonal environment domain, factors such as social support and environmental barriers are critical to take into consideration as Shirley attempts to make meaning of her situation (Elliot et al., 2002). The relationship between social support and PTG has been well documented among trauma populations (Prati & Pietrantoni, 2009). In the initial aftermath of a traumatic event or adjusting to chronic disability, Shirley's use of former friends and a faith context will provide social support.

The use of religious coping and turning to a higher power may also aid in the adjustment process among populations with chronic illness and disability (Kaye & Raghavan, 2002). A clinician should assess patients' spiritual and religious commitments, and when appropriate make referrals to connect individuals with spiritual and religious services. Also, it may be helpful to assess the degree to which one's spiritual beliefs have been challenged by an event, since it is not uncommon for individuals to ask "why did God let this happen to me." Spiritual and religious support was essential for Shirley to remain united and connected with a higher power, in a time when she felt totally disconnected from other persons.

Peer support programs have been used to aid in positive adjustment following TBIs (Hanks et al., 2012) and SCIs (Balcazar, Kelly, Keys, & Balfanz-Vertiz, 2011). Clinicians may have the opportunity to connect patients with peer support programs or with individuals who have gone through similar challenging events. Research suggests that coming into contact with a growth model, or someone who has experienced growth, may also lead to growth (Cobb, Tedeschi, Calhoun, & Cann, 2006).

Along with peer support, engagement in leisure activities promotes growth among individuals with SCIs. The engagement in leisure activities that are meaning based is especially important for individuals adjusting to their new lives and disability as these activities provide opportunities to identify personal strength, build companionship, make sense of their injury, and generate positive emotions (Chun & Lee, 2010).

Although this chapter has focused on the individual who has experienced the new onset disability, clinicians also work closely with family members during the recovery and rehabilitation process. Significant others or caregivers also experience growth from the patients hardship or adversity (e.g., Tallman et al., 2014). Those support persons anticipate, with some degree of accuracy, the amount of growth the patient may experience. Assessing the patient's growth, along with the significant other's perception of the patient's growth, may aid in understanding how growth is occurring within the family system (Berger & Weiss, 2009).

When an individual is completing rehabilitation, it is often away from residence, family, and friends, in an unfamiliar hospital or rehabilitation setting. The unfamiliar place coincides with feelings of uncertainty and ambiguity of making a full recovery, and the perception that one has limited or no control over one's current situation. All of these factors can contribute to the individual experiencing ongoing distress within a rehabilitation environment. Assisting the patient to enhance control and predictability in the environment may help ameliorate the negative adjustment associated with the environment and promote positive coping. Enhancing the perception of predictability and controllability over one's situation may assist individuals in beginning to make sense of their situation, enhancing hope for the future, and creating new goals and life priorities.

The phenomenological and appraisal process domain addresses the appraisal of new stressors (Elliot et al., 2002). Clinicians are in a unique position to understand patients' coping styles (e.g., approach versus avoidance coping) and how different types of coping may be adaptive or maladaptive. Especially in the aftermath of new-onset disability, assessing preexisting strengths and coping styles is paramount. From a clinical standpoint, it is advantageous to understand how the patient has coped with adversity in the past, as this may be an indicator of how they respond or adjust to their new disability. In Shirley's case, medical factors, such as PTA, initially inhibited Shirley's ability to successfully adapt to her spinal cord and traumatic brain injury. As she stabilized medically and psychologically, she used spiritual coping and she began to appraise her situation as manageable. She gained a sense of hope and she gained a fighting spirit.

Early in the rehabilitation process, appraisal and coping processes may manifest in the individual using defensive denial, associated with positive and negative outcomes (Kortte & Wegener, 2004). As mentioned throughout this chapter, the creation of positive illusions or the use of denial may serve a very important purpose in the early stages of adjustment to a newly acquired disability. For example, Shirley believed she would be better off after her accident than before; she believed that she would walk again. It is important to help the patient balance reality with complete denial of the situation. The clinician should, therefore, be willing to accept that the creation of the positive illusion may serve an adaptive purpose. In the initial stages of recovery, it is safer psychologically to believe in partial or full recovery than to fully accept the extent in which one's life has changed forever. The use of denial may serve to enhance hope and motivation, and serve an important role in continuing to participate, meaningfully, in one's recovery and rehabilitation activities. Shirley's thought to "walk out of the hospital" is not likely to happen, but it motivated her engagement in rehabilitation activities. Thus, accepting illusions as helpful and enhancing hope are essential to the patient continuing to deal with their disability.

The psychological well-being and physical health domain encompasses physical and mental health. Although growth tends to be positively linked to distress in the early stages following new-onset disability, this relationship may change over time, with growth being positively linked to adaptive outcomes, over time. If the clinician has the opportunity to work with a patient from the early to late stages of adjusting to the disability, the clinician may see these changes emerge, and assist the patient with formulating new life goals and purpose in life.

CONCLUSIONS AND FUTURE IMPLICATIONS

Although not all individuals experience growth following adversity, our review of the literature suggests that many individuals do experience PTG in the aftermath of SCI, TBI, amputation, pain conditions, cardiac conditions, and other acquired disabilities. Acquiring a disability and learning to adjust to one's new reality creates opportunities for individuals to reprioritize life goals and experience PTG. Clinicians can play a significant role in this process by helping individuals navigate the complex adjustment process. Growth is multidimensional and it may manifest differently at various time points following traumatic events.

As noted, the use of defensive denial, or the creation of positive illusions, may play an important role for someone who struggles with the aftermath of his or her disability. Gaining a greater understanding of this distinction may aid in clinicians differentiating between whether growth is illusory or constructive, which in turn may help the clinician have a clearer conceptualization of the coping process. At a minimum, it is important for clinicians to point out and reflect themes of growth to help individuals come to terms with their situations and their new realities.

Shirley's life was far from normal following her accident. With that said, the meaning that she made and the growth that she perceived allowed her to persevere and go on to live a very normal life with her daughter. She learned to appreciate herself as a person, her strengths and deficits, while accepting her disability and new reality. Her closeness with her daughter was stronger than it had ever been, along with her belief in God. She was able to find hope and learn how to manage the physical and psychological consequences of her disability. She was able to move forward in her life and create a new narrative.

REFERENCES

Americans with disabilities Act of 1990. Pub. L. No. 101-336, 104 Stat. 328 (1990).

Asbring, P. (2001). Chronic illness – a disruption in life: identity-transformation among women with chronic fatigue syndrome and fibromyalgia. *Journal of Advanced Nursing, 34*(3), 312–319. http://dx.doi.org/10.1046/j.1365-2648.2001.01767.x.

Baillie, S. E., Sellwood, W., & Wisely, J. A. (2014). Post-traumatic growth in adults following a burn. *Burns: Journal of the International Society for Burn Injuries, 40,* 1089–1096. http://dx.doi.org/10.1016/j.burns.2014.04.007.

Balcazar, F. E., Kelly, E. H., Keys, C. B., & Balfanz-Vertiz, K. (2011). Using peer mentoring to support the rehabilitation of individuals with violently acquired spinal cord injuries. *Journal of Applied Rehabilitation Counseling, 42*(4), 3.

Benetato, B. B. (2011). Posttraumatic growth among operation enduring freedom and operation Iraqi freedom amputees. *Journal of Nursing Scholarship, 43*(4), 412–420. http://dx.doi.org/10.1111/j.1547-5069.2011.01421.x.

Berger, R., & Weiss, T. (2009). The Posttraumatic Growth model: an expansion to the family system. *Traumatology, 15*(1), 63–74. http://dx.doi.org/10.1177/1534765608323499.

Boerner, K., & Wang, S. W. (2010). How it matters when it happens: life changes related to functional loss in younger and older adults. *The International Journal of Aging and Human Development, 70*(2), 163–179. http://dx.doi.org/10.2190/ag.70.2.

Boerner, K., Wang, S., & Cimarolli, V. R. (2006). The impact of functional loss: nature and implications of life changes. *Journal of Loss and Trauma, 11,* 265–287. http://dx.doi.org/10.1080/15325020600066262.

Bombardier, C. H., Ehde, D. M., Stoelb, B., & Molton, I. R. (2010). The relationship of age-related factors to psychological functioning among people with disabilities. *Physical Medicine and Rehabilitation Clinics of North America, 21*(2), 281–297. http://dx.doi.org/10.1016/j.pmr.2009.12.005.

Bonanno, G. A. (2004). Loss, trauma, and human resilience: have we underestimated the human capacity to thrive after extremely aversive events. *American Psychologist, 59,* 20–28. http://dx.doi.org/10.1037/0003-066x.59.1.20.

Bonanno, G. A., Westphal, M., & Mancini, A. D. (2011). Resilience to loss and potential trauma. *Annual Review of Clinical Psychology, 7,* 511–535.

Brault, M. W. (2012). http://dx.doi.org/10.1146/annurev-clinpsy-032210-104526.

Calhoun, L. G., & Tedeschi, R. G. (2012). Facilitating posttraumatic growth through expert companionship. In L. G. Calhoun, & R. G. Tedeschi (Eds.), *Posttraumatic growth in clinical practice* (pp. 23–38). New York, NY: Routledge.

Chun, S., & Lee, Y. (2010). The role of leisure in the experience of posttraumatic growth for people with spinal cord injury. *Journal of Leisure Research, 42*(3), 393–415.

Cobb, A. R., Tedeschi, R. G., Calhoun, L. G., & Cann, A. (2006). Correlates of posttraumatic growth in survivors of intimate partner violence. *Journal of Traumatic Stress, 19*(6), 895–903. http://dx.doi.org/10.1002/jts.20171.

Cordova, M. J., Cunningham, L. L. C., Carlson, C. R., & Andrykowski, M. A. (2001). Post-traumatic growth following breast cancer: a controlled comparison study. *Health Psychology, 20,* 176–185. http://dx.doi.org/10.1037/0278-6133.20.3.176.

Danoff-Burg, S., & Revenson, T. A. (2005). Benefit-finding among patients with rheumatoid arthritis: positive effects on interpersonal relationships. *Journal of Behavioral Medicine, 28*(1), 91–103. http://dx.doi.org/10.1007/s10865-005-2720-3.

Dembo, T., Leviton, G. L., & Wright, B. A. (1956). Adjustment to misfortune—a problem of social-psychological rehabilitation. *Artificial Limbs, 3*(2), 4–62. http://dx.doi.org/10.1037/h0090832.

Dunn, D. S. (1996). Well-being following amputation: Salutary effects of positive meaning, optimism, and control. *Rehabilitation Psychology, 41,* 285–302.

Dunn, D. S., & Dougherty, S. B. (2005). Prospects for a positive psychology of rehabilitation. *Rehabilitation Psychology, 50*(3), 305. http://dx.doi.org/10.1037/0090-5550.50.3.305.

Dunn, D. S., Uswatte, G., Elliott, T. R., Lastres, A., & Beard, B. (2013). A Positive psychology of physical disability: principles and progress. In *The Oxford handbook of positive psychology and disability* (pp. 427).

Ehde, D. M. (2010). Application of positive psychology to rehabilitation psychology. *Handbook of Rehabilitation Psychology, 2,* 417–424.

Elliott, T. R., Kurylo, M., & Rivera, P. (2002). Positive growth following acquired physical disability. *Handbook of Positive Psychology,* 687–699.

Elliott, T. R., & Richards, J. S. (1999). Living with the facts, negotiating the terms: unrealistic beliefs, denial, and adjustment in the first year of acquired physical disability. *Journal of Personal & Interpersonal Loss, 4*(4), 361–381.

Fredrickson, B. L. (2001). The role of positive emotions in positive psychology: the broaden-and-build theory of positive emotions. *American psychologist, 56*(3), 218.

Gallant, M. P. (2003). The influence of social support on chronic illness self-management: a review and directions for research. *Health Education & Behavior, 30*(2), 170–195.

Gangstad, B., Norman, P., & Barton, J. (2009). Cognitive processing and posttraumatic growth after stroke. *Rehabilitation Psychology, 54*(1), 69–75. http://dx.doi.org/10.1037/a0014639.

Garnefski, N., Kraaij, V., Schroevers, M. J., & Somsen, G. A. (2008). Post-traumatic growth after a myocardial infarction: a matter of personality, psychological health, or cognitive coping? *Journal of Clinical Psychology in Medical Settings, 15,* 270–277. http://dx.doi.org/10.1007/s10880-008-9136-5.

Hanks, R. A., Rapport, L. J., Wertheimer, J., & Koviak, C. (2012). Randomized controlled trial of peer mentoring for individuals with traumatic brain injury and their significant others. *Archives of Physical Medicine and Rehabilitation, 93*(8), 1297–1304.

Hefferon, K., Grealy, M., & Mutrie, N. (2009). Post-traumatic growth and life threatening physical illness: a systematic review of the qualitative literature. *British Journal of Health Psychology, 14*(2), 343–378.

Helgeson, V. S., Reynolds, K. A., & Tomich, P. L. (2006). A meta-analytic review of benefit finding and growth. *Journal of Consulting and Clinical Psychology, 74*(5), 797.

Kaye, J., & Raghavan, S. K. (2002). Spirituality in disability and illness. *Journal of Religion and Health, 41*(3), 231–242.

Kennedy, P., Marsh, N., Lowe, R., Grey, N., Short, E., & Rogers, B. (2000). A longitudinal analysis of psychological impact and coping strategies following spinal cord injury. *British Journal of Health Psychology, 5*(2), 157–172.

Kortte, K. B., & Wegener, S. T. (2004). Denial of illness in medical rehabilitation populations: theory, research, and definition. *Rehabilitation Psychology, 49*(3), 187.

Krause, J. S., & Rohe, D. E. (1998). Personality and life adjustment after spinal cord injury: an exploratory study. *Rehabilitation Psychology, 43*(2), 118.

Lazarus, R. S., & Folkman, S. (1984). *Stress. Appraisal, and coping*, 725.

Leung, Y. W., Gravely-Witte, S., Macpherson, A., & Irvine, J. (2010). Post-traumatic growth among cardiac outpatients. Degree comparison with other chronic illness samples and correlates. *Journal of Health Psychology, 15*(7), 1049–1063. http://dx.doi.org/10.1177/1359105309360577.

Luttik, M. L., Jaarsma, T., Moser, D., Sanderman, R., & van Veldhuisen, D. J. (2005). The importance and impact of social support on outcomes in patients with heart failure: an overview of the literature. *Journal of Cardiovascular Nursing, 20*(3), 162–169.

Oaksford, R., Frude, N., & Cuddihy, R. (2005). Positive coping and stress-related psychological growth following lower-limb amputation. *Rehabilitation Psychology, 50*, 266–277.

Phelps, L. F., Williams, R. M., Raichle, K. A., Turner, A. P., & Ehde, D. M. (2008). The importance of cognitive processing to adjustment in the 1st year following amputation. *Rehabilitation Psychology, 53*(1), 28–38. http://dx.doi.org/10.1037/0090-5550.53.1.28.

Pollard, C., & Kennedy, P. (2007). A longitudinal analysis of emotional impact, coping strategies and post-traumatic psychological growth following spinal cord injury: a 10-year review. *British Journal of Health Psychology, 12*, 347–362. http://dx.doi.org/10.1348/135910707X197046.

Powell, T., Gilson, R., & Collin, C. (2012). TBI 13 years on: factors associated with post-traumatic growth. *Disability and Rehabilitation, 34*(17), 1461–1467.

Prati, G., & Pietrantoni, L. (2009). Optimism, social support, and coping strategies as factors contributing to posttraumatic growth: a meta-analysis. *Journal of Loss and Trauma, 14*(5), 364–388.

Roepke, A. M. (2015). Psychosocial interventions and posttraumatic growth: a meta-analysis. *Journal of Clinical and Consulting Psychology, 83*, 129–142.

Rogan, C., Fortune, D. G., & Prentice, G. (2013). Post-traumatic growth, illness perceptions and coping in people with acquired brain injury. *Neuropsychological Rehabilitation: An International Journal, 23*(5), 639–657. http://dx.doi.org/10.1080/09602011.2013.799076.

Rosenbach, C., & Renneberg, B. (2008). Positive change after severe burn injuries. *Journal of Burn Care & Research, 29*(4), 638–643. http://dx.doi.org/10.1097/BCR.0b013e31817de275.

Salick, E. C., & Auerbach, C. F. (2006). From devastation to integration: adjusting to and growing from medical trauma. *Qualitative Health Research, 16*(8), 1021–1037.

Seligman, M. E. P., & Csikszentmihalyi, M. (2000). Positive psychology: an introduction. *American Psychologist, 55*, 5–14.

Silva, J., Ownsworth, T., Shields, C., & Fleming, J. (2011). Enhanced appreciation of life following acquired brain injury: posttraumatic growth at 6 months postdischarge. *Brain Impairment, 12*(2), 93–104. http://dx.doi.org/10.1375/brim.12.2.93.

Snyder, C. R. (1989). Reality negotiation: from excuses to hope and beyond. *Journal of Social and Clinical Psychology, 8*, 130–157.

Tallman, B. A. (2013). Anticipated posttraumatic growth from cancer: the roles of adaptive and maladaptive coping strategies. *Counselling Psychology Quarterly, 26*(1), 72–88.

Tallman, B. A., Lohnberg, J., Yamada, T. H., Halfdanarson, T. R., & Altmaier, E. M. (2014). Anticipating posttraumatic growth from cancer: patients' and collaterals' experiences. *Journal of Psychosocial Oncology, 32*(3), 342–358.

Tedeschi, R. G., & Calhoun, L. G. (1996). Posttraumatic growth inventory: measuring the positive legacy of trauma. *Journal of Traumatic Stress, 9*, 455–471.

Tedeschi, R. G., & Calhoun, L. G. (2004). Posttraumatic growth: conceptual foundations and empirical evidence. *Psychological Inquiry, 15*, 1–18.

Tedeschi, R. G., & Calhoun, L. G. (2009). The clinician as expert companion. In C. L. Park, S. C. Lechner, M. H. Antoni, & A. L. Stanton (Eds.), *Medical illness and positive life change: Can crisis lead to personal transformation?* (pp. 215–235) Washington, DC: APA.

Tedeschi, R. G., & McNally, R. J. (2011). Can we facilitate posttraumatic growth in combat veterans? *American Psychologist, 66*, 19–24. http://dx.doi.org/10.1037/a0021896.

Tuncay, T., & Musabak, I. (2015). Problem-focused coping strategies predict posttraumatic growth in veterans with lower-limb amputations. *Journal of Social Service Research.* http://dx.doi.org/10.1080/01488376.2015.1033584.

Wehmeyer, M. L. (2013). *The oxford handbook of positive psychology and disability.* Oxford University Press.

Weiss, T., & Berger, R. (Eds.). (2010). *Posttraumatic growth and culturally competent practice: Lessons learned from around the globe.* Hoboken, NJ: Wiley.

Widows, M. R., Jacobsen, P. B., Booth-Jones, M., & Fields, K. K. (2005). Predictors of posttraumatic growth following bone marrow transplantation for cancer. *Health Psychology, 24*(3), 266.

Wright, B. A. P. (1983). *Physical disability, a psychosocial approach.* New York, NY: Harper & Row, Publisher, Inc.

Wright, B. A. (1989). Extension of Heider's ideas to rehabilitation psychology. *American Psychologist, 44,* 525–528.

Zoellner, T., & Maercker, A. (2006). Posttraumatic growth in clinical psychology—A critical review and introduction of a two component model. *Clinical Psychology Review, 26*(5), 626–653.

CHAPTER 10

Expressive Arts: A Group Intervention for Unaccompanied Minor Asylum Seekers and Young Adults

M.A. Meyer DeMott[1,2,3]
[1]University College of South East Norway, Oslo, Norway; [2]Norwegian Institute for Expressive Arts and Communications, Oslo, Norway; [3]European Graduate School, Saas Fee, Switzerland

"Elisabeth," a refugee from Turkey, experienced the images she created and shaped as more powerful than words. Elisabeth said:

I experienced drawing as very helpful. When I draw, I don't control. When the control is gone, you come direct to the core of the issue, sorrow, happiness - whatever it is. Words are very limited. I found words through the images I drew. It is the images that make the words meaningful, not the words that make the image work.

What I remember best is an image I drew: There are many women wearing black clothes and a war is going on. The women are carrying water and it's very quiet. It's a place where everything is left in ruins. Children are crying and the women are in deep sorrow. It is as though this picture is from an earlier life. I am stuck with this image.

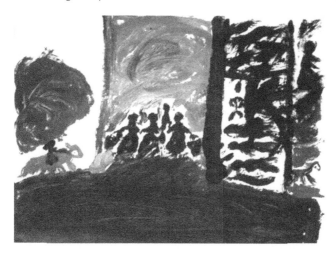

Reconstructing Meaning After Trauma
ISBN 978-0-12-803015-8
http://dx.doi.org/10.1016/B978-0-12-803015-8.00010-3

Here I am riding through the dry landscape, it is warm and the dust whirls up all around me. The women are carrying their babies, children walk alongside. Everything is happening on the same earth, Mother Earth. Death, corpses, funerals, grief, aggression, if only I could get back on the horse's back, so the journey could continue. But I am stuck in the grief. I am stuck with the sadness and losses that were awakened in prison - the losses in my childhood, the feeling of loneliness, despair, hopelessness, powerlessness. If I get back on my horse's back I may just ride in a circle and have to go through it all over again.

I asked her how this image makes her feel.

I feel pain. I experience the sorrow and the stillness. The women are patient, they are coping and supporting each other without saying anything. They have been very patient. I have respect for these women. They are wise and strong.

Maybe this picture is stuck in Elisabeth's mind because it connects her to the life and stories of many. Elisabeth belonged to a revolutionary party. The family was poor and lived in a small village. Her mother died when she was age 8 years. At the age of 17 years, she was arrested and sent to prison. Her sister and brother were tortured in front of her while she was interrogated. Her father died while she was in prison. At the age of 21 years, after 4 years in prison, she managed to escape. She was given the status of political refugee after 3 years in a reception center in Norway. She participated in the Expressive Arts (EXA) group at the Psychosocial Centre for Refugees (Meyer, 2004).

EXPRESSIVE ARTS

In EXA a therapist uses various expressive modalities. EXA considers non-verbal forms of expression to be an essential part of the human being's total communication, including expressions through and from the body. EXA involves a combination of movement, visual art, music, poetry, drama, and film. The intermodal approach builds on the understanding that all expressions are body based and connected to the senses.

The therapist selects the art sensory modality that is most adequate for the client's need for expression, and emotional investigation. The intermodal approach adds one expressive modality to another, touching all venues of human communication from and within the body. The process of creation is emphasized, rather than the final product.

EXA therapy is based on the assumption that people can heal through the use of imagination, physical and mental movement, connection, playing, being present, and the various forms of creative expression.

Paolo Knill is the "founder" of Intermodal Expressive Arts Therapy. He created a theory of practice. The theory was shaped and documented in

Principles and Practice of Expressive Arts Therapy (Knill, Levine, & Levine, 2005). Knill's "crystallization theory" (Knill, Barba, & Fuchs, 1995; Knill, 1999) is an important element in Expressive Arts Therapy, an integrated, independent arts-based psychotherapy based on a phenomenological philosophy and attitude toward life. "The theory attempts to formulate how the helping relationship can provide optimal conditions for emerging images to come to their potential through the use of different art disciplines" (Knill et al., 2005, p. 123).

The arts communicate from the senses to the senses. Intermodal transfer is when we change from one art modality to a new one—creating a poem to the image, creating music to the poem, movement to the music. In this way, we involve all the senses and stay with the image. Intermodal transfer gives new perspectives of the image without moving into the literate reality. We stay with the concreteness of the art experience before we go to the depth. We communicate with the image using all our senses, trying to make sense out of our experiences with the help of our imagination.

As a parallel, play has no beginning or end. It involves all the senses and demands total presence. Play is the opposite of a game where rules and goals are defined and participants either win or lose. EXA operates with "the liminal" process, where one is not clear about what the outcome will be. The participants do not have to have the skills or the talents of an artist. Many have not touched a paintbrush since they were children. Communicating with a different and unfamiliar medium can give new perspectives.

"Habitual worlding" (Knill et al., 2005: 85–90) is the way we exist in the world out of habit. What we do habitually are routines or rituals we do every day consciously or unconsciously, like going to the bathroom, eating, sleeping, going to school, all events that we are not necessarily conscious of. Habitual worlding is a person's narrative out of habit; the way he or she normally communicates oneself to the world. If life only consisted of habitual worlding, it would be a passive way of living where imagination and the act of creating were missing.

"Alternative worlding" is doing something different from the normal routine, communicating with the world in a new way. Alternative worlding is using a new narrative genre to tell a person's story—playing with the story, shaping it, and reshaping it (Knill et al., 2005). Alternative worlding is a spontaneous and creative act. To be able to become spontaneous again, it is necessary to be distanced from the conflict. This action is called decentering. You create a play space—where the participants distant themselves from the conflict by making art that demands total presence in the here and now.

The arts open the senses. We touch each other by seeing, hearing, moving, and feeling. The artwork is the main form of communication in EXA therapy. Storytelling through the performing arts is practiced all over the world and is one of the oldest traditions in human history. Today when populations are becoming less homogenous it is important that therapeutic approaches try to build bridges between people and cultures. An excellent example are the theorists and practitioners in Scandinavia, who have made contributions to the EXA field (see Meyer, 1995, 1999, 2004; Meyer DeMott, 1999, 2007, 2014; Ødegaard & Meyer DeMott, 2008; Stubbe, 2011; Wärja, 2004).

EXA GROUPS AND RECONSTRUCTING MEANING AFTER TRAUMA

Traumatic experiences such as suicide bombings, torture, and organized violence have an enormous impact on the senses. The normal reaction is to shut down, to protect oneself from these overwhelming impressions. The senses shut down. What made sense before becomes senseless.

It is worth noting, however, that in a prison camp being "bodily dead" can function as a defense mechanism. To endure an intolerable situation, the functioning of the senses is reduced, thus limiting the ability of sensing feelings, such as anger and fear. Going into "exile" from the body can be a way of protecting the "self" from being totally destroyed. Pain, humiliation, and powerlessness are minimized by not being present.

When a mouse is being tortured by a cat, the mouse "plays dead," hoping that the cat will lose interest and leave. Similarly, being "bodily dead" might make a person less likely to be tortured. The closer a person is to death, the more he or she will be left alone mentally and physically, so in this context the "bodily dead" state of being can be a positive factor.

People who have survived trauma often express that they have no words, that they have lost their language. They feel like they have fallen apart. Who am I now? What will I become? The survivor is in a "liminal" space, not being who she or he was and not knowing what to become. Finding expression for what they yet do not have words helps to shape new meaning. "Within a therapeutic context, artistic creativity can itself be understood as a form of soul-making which aims to restore sense to the world" (Levine, 2009, p. 45). In other words, meaning is created from shaping and reshaping in artistic expressions from the senseless and wordless experiences. By giving these experiences a shape they become visible and can help to reconnect the survivor to the world.

Imagination is the bridge from the internal to the external world (Winnicott, 1971). In a healthy person, this relationship between inner and outer world, between fantasy and imagination, is a dialectical one, constantly moving. After trauma, the relationship is often deadlocked. The "play space" is the "transitional space" and gives the survivor of trauma the opportunity to get "unlocked" and free.

Winnicott states that when children start playing again after a traumatic experience, it means they have bounced back. They use their senses to navigate their way back to their childhood and to play. Play is a form of communication; it is relational and can imply trust. It is also about producing, shaping, and transforming something. This activity relates to using imagination and creativity that ultimately can enhance their identity and increase their range of play.

Being in exile is potentially a traumatic experience. It interrupts the sense of "going on being" and breaks the frame of reference that is provided by one's cultural codes. It causes regression, which takes the person back into the stage of "formlessness" (Winnicott, 1971).

In EXA we shape and reshape until the "formlessness" has found a form. Through the process of reshaping meaning can emerge again.

Ibrahim, a Bosnian refugee who participated in a movement group at the arrival center Fossnes in Norway, said:

> For four to five months, moving around was forbidden in the concentration camp. Our hands were tied behind our backs. We could not move our heads; we were only allowed to look down. Of course, the movement program was such a relief after all of this. Everybody who has been in a concentration camp, not only in Manjaca where I was, should be advised to participate in the movement program, because everybody there lied on a concrete floor without being allowed to move and was not able to use their voice or their body. Gymnastics in the Norwegian way helps improve your health very much. It doesn't only give bodily relief but also relieves the soul – both in the lungs and in the thoughts. Yes, the exercises with breathing deep in and out. We had gymnastics earlier in school, but never in this way.

Meyer (1995), Meyer DeMott (2007, p. 54) and Meyer DeMott (1996).

After an experience like a concentration camp, people become fragmented and depressed—they lose sense and meaning. Instead of looking for new images, hearing the present music, smelling the scent of the flowers, and feeling the joy of being alive, the senses become locked to the traumatic events. The Bosnian refugees could not find words. But through movement, they were able to express emotions and images. Paolo Knill says that each art discipline is a vehicle for the imagination. "One can be moved through music, a story, or a scene, or one can describe motion pictures, but most certainly movement is experienced strongly through its crystallization in dance. There is no dance, mime etc., without movement" (2005, p. 123). Working with the arts can help the participants to create a new way of communicating and help them to see, hear, and sense each other, not only the "demons from the past." van der Kolk and van der Hart (1991) said that memory is flexible, but when it gets attached to one traumatic image, it loses its role of restoring balance in the psyche.

In his book *Testimony* (Felman/Laub, 1992), Dori Laub refers to the "I witness," the witness within, and the "outer witness," the witness to the world. The trauma survivor is often stuck with trying to communicate exactly what happened and this is a trap many trauma survivors never escape. The witness in the world can never perceive the event exactly the way it happened. The witness in the world can imagine what it was like through his or her life experiences and creativity.

STUCK TO THE MEMORY OF ONE IMAGE

Many clients who suffer from chronic posttraumatic stress disorder (PTSD) are persecuted by certain traumatic events. These memories represent a threat of some kind, for instance, no place to go, no place to hide, no exit, and so on. Are these images declarative, representing one specific event, or symbolic for the state of being alive? The images certainly illustrate the problem, but are not literate. They are created with help of the imagination. Elisabeth said that she thought maybe the picture came from a past life. Maybe we all have one image that tells "the whole story"? What these unique images have in common is that they carry not only the suffering but also the yearning it is calling for. Is the soul trying to send a message? What is the soul asking for? Shall we play more with these images, identify them earlier and play with them, or should we abandon them and move on?

It is important to abandon the literate trauma story and not try to communicate the event through one art form but through several. Here, intermodal transfer helps the survivor to work with the senses and gain new perspectives. Going to a new media together with the witness and beginning to use the imagination to create a new "story," which also includes the images of the witness, functions as a bridge to the world out of isolation and gives a sense of being seen and touched by one another. Working with the arts activates all the senses and gives an experience of being alive in the moment. What was senseless makes sense, in the art making one can find meaning.

65 MILLION REFUGEES

As of the writing of this chapter, we are experiencing the largest refugee crises since World War 2. In 2016, we reached a new record of 65 million (Norwegian Refugee Council, 2016). In 2015 about 38 million refugees were internally displaced and the majority came from Syria (6.5 million). Being a refugee challenges the organism both physically and mentally. The individual is disconnected, rejected, unsafe, and in doubt about the future. It is estimated that one half of the total refugee population are children. They are the most vulnerable group and the largest concern for the High Commissioner of Refugees (UNHCR). Over the past 3 years, 12,000 children have been killed in Syria, an average of 12 per day. The act of war has changed from being one state against another to civil wars where civilians and children often are legitimate targets. They are forced to escape and live in exile.

What Does It Mean to Live in Exile?

Exile is often reported as a more devastating experience than torture and is a new trauma on top of the old. Exile is here defined in four different categories:

1. **Political exile.** The refugees' perception is not congruent with the government in their mother country. The extension of their punishment is that they are not welcome in their own country.
2. **Emotional exile.** They can come home according to the government, but because of going through radical culture differences while living in exile, they feel it emotionally impossible to return. Children risk being mobbed because they have become so different while they lived in exile. Another example is a man who felt he could not return to Chile because when he was in exile and the police failed to find him, they tortured his brother instead.
3. **Exile from the body.** Refugees live "outside of their bodies" and observe the body as though it were someone else's. This coping mechanism of dissociating from the body is one of the most common among torture victims. Their bodies are numb and they have no emotional affect.
4. **Exile from culture.** Refugees come from cultures that are radically different from the new country's in language, religion, climate, and social interaction. They are living outside of their culture.

Living in exile in addition to previous traumas can lead to isolation, lack of self-esteem, apathy, numbness, depression, and guilt (Meyer DeMott, 2007).

Since refugees have already lost so much, they are afraid of getting attached and having to go through the pain of separating again. It is better to stay isolated and live in a vacuum than engage in the present and look to the future. Living in a different culture breaks the continuity in one's life. Also, most refugees come from countries where it is dangerous to express one's opinion. For example, in their school they are expected to learn what the textbook and teacher says. In the new environment, they are encouraged to think for themselves, and teaching often occurs in group discussions. This change can be very threatening for someone who has lived with the fear of being killed for expressing him or herself.

Living in exile means that you are living involuntarily in a country. You cannot leave if you do not like the food, the weather, the music, or the politics. It is a totally different experience than when you know that you are only going to stay temporarily and have a date for returning home. The longer you live in exile, the smaller the probability is that you will ever be able to return home, so even refugees who can go home feel that they cannot for many different reasons. They have changed and the country they left has changed.

THE THERAPEUTIC FACTORS OF EXA GROUPS WORKING WITH TRAUMA SURVIVORS LIVING IN EXILE

Judith Lewis Herman says in *Trauma and recovery* (1992) that one of the most important treatments for people suffering from trauma and PTSD is group therapy. But the factors that allow a group to function and not collapse can be very demanding for the same reasons why group therapy is so important. The most challenging symptoms are lack of trust in other people, withdrawal, depression, low presence, distorted identity, and no sense of time. All these symptoms make it difficult for the trauma survivors to connect. Arriving in a new land brings up anxieties of the unknown and therefore causes regression, which can either be a malign one or a benign one that will lead to a new beginning (Balint, 1968). "Perhaps this is the time when playing, for the second time in an immigrant's life, has the utmost importance, because once more he has to be able to play in order to create a new 'bicultural self'" (Sengun, 2001, p.71). The arts create a bridge between the participants—they connect and engage through "the third"—the arts.

Yalom (1975) divides the therapeutic factors of group psychotherapy into 11 primary categories:

1. Installation of hope—knowing that other people have similar experiences and problems.
2. Universality—my experiences are similar to the rest of the group.

3. Imparting of information—sharing stories and images with the other members.
4. Altruism—by helping another I help myself.
5. The corrective recapitulation of the primary family group—I can be part of a family, a group in the future.
6. Development of socializing techniques—breaking the isolation and bonding with others.
7. Imitative behavior—being role models for each other. If you can, so can I.
8. Interpersonal learning—identifying resources in the individual and in the group.
9. Group cohesiveness—being received and respected and receiving and respecting others.
10. Catharsis—learning how to cope and express difficult feelings in the presence of others.
11. Existential factors—dealing with existential problems and exploring the future.

Based on an EXA group research project with torture survivors carried out at the Psychosocial Centre for Refugees in Oslo, Norway, in 1993–2000, we found that EXA adds eight more therapeutic factors (Meyer, 2004). These factors emerged from the experiences of the participants with the EXA methods. These methods enhanced the group's resources and we could identify them and use them in communicating with each other:

1. Being treated as an individual with an identity, instead of being an object.
2. Identifying the resources in the group through art making.
3. The arts can help the clients find an expression for their symptoms and learn to cope with the symptoms with the help of each other.
4. Being in the present, in the here and now.
5. The group functions as a witness to each member's testimony.
6. Movement creates energy and gives a sense of life in the body.
7. Through the arts, the group will gain new perspectives.
8. Artmaking is distancing and gives permission to play in the transitional space. Creating group rituals helps restore psychological balance.

In the interviews I asked: "When you think of the group what do you remember?"

"Imir" answered:

It was the most important day of the week to come and participate in the group.

For me it was important to come to the group. When I came here I did not feel alone with my problems. The people around me had similar problems. I felt a freedom to speak about my experiences without being labeled as crazy or looked down on.

Hobfoll et al. (2007) studied early intervention after mass trauma and concluded: "Given the devastation caused by disasters and mass violence it is critical that intervention policy be based on the most updated research findings. However, to date, no evidence-based consensus has been reached supporting a clear set of recommendations for intervention during the immediate and mid-term mass trauma phases (p. 283–284)." A worldwide panel of experts on the study and treatment of those exposed to disaster and mass violence was assembled to extrapolate from related fields of research, and to gain consensus on intervention principles. They identified five empirically supported intervention principles that should be used to guide and inform intervention and prevention efforts at the early to mid-term stages. These are promoting a sense of safety, calming, a sense of self- and community efficacy, connectedness, and hope.

The EXA group in a very basic way gives the feeling of being connected with others, which is important for the refugee who has lost his connection with his own country, people, and culture. It supports and strengthens the capacity to be alone. It also gives a sense of continuity and hence a feeling of security. The group is a place where the patient has a sense of "going on being" (Sengun, 2001).

Based on this research, an early intervention study was developed: Expressive Arts in Transition (EXIT) (Meyer DeMott, 2014). EXIT is a short term, component-based group intervention. EXIT requires active participation and integrates interpersonal, cognitive, and behavior-oriented interventions. The target sample were boys between 15 and 18 years newly arrived at the Hvalstad Arrival Centre for unaccompanied asylum seeking children (UASC). A research assistant working at Hvalstad invited all minors who arrived in certain periods (12 weeks in 2009, 8 weeks in 2010, and 13 weeks in 2011) to participate in the study. Only UASC boys were invited since at that time they far outnumbered UASC girls, by 87% to 12.5% in 2009 (Eide & Broch, 2010), and boys were the least studied. Because of the costs of translation and screening instrument testing, only the six largest language groups were selected (Arabic, Dari, Farsi, Somali, Sorani, and Pashto), representing approximately 50% of the total number of asylum-seeking UASC in Norway at the time (2008–2010). To be eligible for the study, the youth had to be willing to stay at Hvalstad for 6 weeks. A total of 71 boys participated in the EXIT group. On arrival 40% had enough posttraumatic stress symptoms to qualify for PTSD (Vervliet et al., 2014). Over a period of two and a half years, the EXIT group showed a decrease in posttraumatic stress, anxiety, and depression. In addition, their quality of life increased and they became more optimistic about the future (Meyer DeMott, 2014).

Many of the refugee boys had similar stories when they arrived. They did not know what countries they had travelled through. Many had been in containers or hidden under trucks for days and weeks. The EXIT workshop consisted of 10 twice-weekly sessions, each lasting 1.5 h. The workshop gave the participants skills for coping with the normal symptoms of stress: sleeplessness, headaches, lack of concentration, irritability, and withdrawal. The first five sessions focused on:

1. Welcome dance: leading and following each other's movements.
2. Imagining and creating a safe place.
3. Future projection: what will you be doing 5 years from today? Move from one end of the room (here and now) to the other end (5 years ahead in time).
4. Finding your inner resource animal. Find its movements and sounds. Dance the animal's dance and have the rest of the group mirror the movements and sounds.
5. Hello and goodbye ritual. Five new participants begin and five leave.

The same structure is repeated in sessions 6–10. We called it the "train model"—five new participants come on board and five participants get off at session 5. This helped to prepare participants for the many beginnings and endings they will experience as asylum seekers.

In EXIT the point of reference is everything that is usually done during the day, all the daily routines. We promoted more awareness of these daily routines: how do you get up in the morning and how do you go to bed—in other words, how do you start and end the day? Routines are rituals that can provide safety and become something predictable in an otherwise unpredictable situation. They can also become a container for pain. Rituals may be divided into four phases: preparation or warming up, action, closure, and a reflection/harvesting phase. All individuals have their own rhythms.

The intervention EXIT functioned as a toolkit for life while the refugees were in the process of applying for asylum and adjusting to a new culture. The activities gave meaning while waiting.

"Amid" from Afghanistan said:

I liked the EXIT group. It did me good. The physical exercises helped against insomnia. When I can't sleep the exercises help me to relax. Because of the program my time in the reception centre became meaningful. We danced and did exercises that helped us.

"Amal" from Somalia:

When we came to Hvalstad Reception centre, we had no family there or in Norway. But we got you and the EXIT group. That helped. Some of us say that you became our new family (Skagen & Meyer DeMott, 2014).

Interventions that can help the refugees in the first phase are group work, helping them connect to themselves and each other. In addition to safety, calming, engaging, efficacy, and hope, the focus is on movement, playing, bodywork, and testimony through movement. The therapist has a psychoeducative approach, teaching the participants to help themselves, to reconnect with their identity before captivity and focus on their resources for survival. It is essential that participants be and feel respected and accepted, not once, not twice, but all the time. The groups can function as a reception ritual. This is community art that is designed with a repetitious beginning and end: creating predictability within the unpredictable is essential.

THE ROLE OF THE THERAPIST

How do you create an atmosphere for healing in a group? Therapy aims to restore the person to the ground of human existence, to the experience of embodied being in the world with others. We could therefore describe therapy as "a rite of restoration" (Knill et al., 2005). The circle is the holding body of the group. In EXA therapy, the response the listener gives to the traumatic stories is called an "aesthetic response." When the story is communicated through art, the witness is able to identify with the story through the body. "The response has a bodily origin. When the response is profound and soul-stirring, we describe it as moving, touching or breathtaking" (Knill et al., 2005: 137). Paolo Knill refers to Gendlin (1981) who describes the response toward an image in a therapeutic context: "He calls the phenomenon in his focusing method a felt sense, it occurs when a quite right image emerges, an image that matches and resonates with the psychic condition of the client and evokes an observable response" (Knill et al., 2005: 137).

An aesthetic response signals the significance of what emerges. Here the whole range of artistic work can be found. An aesthetic response can be given as a story, a painting, a dance, a poem. The aesthetic response expresses the stories that are awoken in the listener. Here lies the seed, the possibility, of the "third narrative," which is the narrative that emerges between the person telling the story and the one(s) receiving it. It is no longer only one person's story, but everyone's story. A real intersubjectivity is then strengthened that creates a sense of solidarity in the group. We share something similar and we can express our stories in our own unique way. We find meaning in the meaningless because we can shape, externalize, and share the artistic expression and experience how it moves and inspires others to share their stories.

The arts are expressions powerful enough to become containers for the emotional pain of the client. Instead of the therapist becoming the receiver of the client's projections, the artwork takes on this role. Creating art gives the participants the necessary distance to each other. Through the art, we can imagine how it is to be the other and relate from our own life experiences. If the listener feels forced to listen to the literate trauma story, he or she may feel invaded. As an EXA therapist I always sense the "group body" and ask: "Is this body breathing, is there enough movement and energy, is this body alive and if not what will it take?"

Being a witness to other people's life stories is very enriching, but also challenging. Research shows that having too much empathy or being over engaged with traumatized patients can lead to compassion fatigue. Compassion fatigue drains the therapist's energy and gives the symptoms of burnout; lack of concentration, irritability, insomnia, lack of interest, and prone accident behavior, like cutting yourself with the bread knife because you are not focused on what you are doing.

Maybe the key to the difficult task of witnessing other people's trauma stories depends on your own research on what you have witnessed inside yourself? Referring to what Dori Laub calls the "I witness": When I hear someone's story, what story is awakened in my life? Maybe you have to make your own life story available and have to experience playing with it? Then you can imagine where your life meets others and provide a safe playing space, a garden where there is room for praise and lament. The plants in the garden must be cared for and the uniqueness of each plant must be respected. Together they create a garden where all can grow. The therapist is the gardener who cares for this unique culture and has the humbleness and strength to take part in creating it. In the garden you will discover new meaning.

REFERENCES

Balint, M. (1968). *The basic fault*. London: Tavistock.
Eide, K., & Broch, T. (2010). *RBUP (Regional centre for youth and Childrens Mental Health) Report*. Oslo Norway.
Felman, S., & Laub, D. (1992). *Testimony*. New York: Routledge.
Herman, J. L. (1992). *Trauma and recovery*. New York: Basic Books.
Hobfoll, S. E., Watson, P., Bell, C. C., Bryant, R. A., Brymer, M. J., Friedman, M. J., ... Ursano, R. J. (2007). Five essential elements of immediate and mid-term mass trauma intervention: imperical evidence. *Psychiatry*, 70(4).
Knill, P. J. (1999). Das Kristallisationsprinzip in einer musikorientierten Musiktherapie. In I. Frohne-Hagemann (Ed.), *Musik und Gestalt. Klinische Musiktherapie als integrative Psychotherapie* (2nd, revised ed.). Göttingen: Vandenhoeck & Ruprecht.

Knill, P. J., Barba, H. N., & Fuchs, M. N. (1995). *Minstrels of soul: intermodal expressive therapy.* Toronto: Palmerstone Press.

Knill, P. J., Levine, E. G., & Levine, S. K. (2005). *Principles and practice of expressive arts therapy. Toward a therapeutic aesthetics.* London: Jessica Kingsley Publishers.

van der Kolk, B. A., & van der Hart, O. (1991). The intrusive past: the flexibility of memory and the engraving of trauma. *American Imago, 48,* 425–454.

Levine, S. K. (2009). *Trauma, tragedy, therapy. The arts and human suffering.* London: Jessica Kingsley Publishers.

Meyer, M. A. (1995). Stress prevention in refugee reception centers. *Energy and Character: The Journal of Biosynthesis, 26*(2), 32–46.

Meyer, M. A. (1999). In exile from the body: creating a play room in the waiting room. In S. K. Levine, & E. G. Levine (Eds.), *Foundations of expressive arts therapy* (pp. 241–255). London: Jessica Kingsley Publishers.

Meyer, M. A. (2004). The garden of praise and lament. *Poiesis, A Journal of the Arts and Communication, 6,* 164–172.

Meyer DeMott, M. A. (1996). *Videofilm: In exile from the body* (21 min) Oslo: Melinda Meyer.

Meyer DeMott, M. A. (1999). *Videofilm: Returning to life* (50 min) Oslo: Melinda Meyer.

Meyer DeMott, M. A. (2007). *Repatriation and testimony. Expressive arts therapy. A phenomenological study of Bosnian war refugees with focus on returning home, testimony and film* (Ph.D. dissertation, Arts, Health & Society Division (EGS)). Switzerland, and Nasjonalt kunnskapssenter om vold og traumatisk stress i Norge. Oslo: Unipub AS.

Meyer DeMott, M. A. (2014). Art as Testimony – Breaking the Silence. In *Do we really Care.* London: Cambridge Scholars Publishing.

Ødegaard, A. J., & Meyer DeMott, M. A. (2008). *Estetisk veiledning. Dialog gjennom kunstuttrykk.* Oslo: Universitetsforlaget.

Sengun, S. (2001). *Migration as a transitional space and group analysis. The group analytical society.* London: SAGE Publications.

Skagen, S., & Meyer DeMott, M. A. (2014). *Videofilm: Exit* (22 min) Oslo: Film & Arts.

Stubbe, H. (2011). Art therapy may reduce psychopathology in schizophrenia by strengthening the patients' sense of self: a qualitative extended case report. *Psychopathology, 44*(5), 314–318.

Vervliet, M., Meyer DeMott, M. A., Jakobsen, M., Broekaert, E., Heir, T., & Derluyn, I. (2014). The mental health of unaccompanied refugee minors on arrival in the host country. *Scandinavian Journal of Psychology, 55,* 33–37.

Wärja, M. (2004). Music as Mother. In S. K. Levine, & E. G. Levine (Eds.), *Foundations of Expressive arts Therapy. Theoretical and Clinical Perspectives* (Vol. 4). London: Jessica Kingsley Publishers (23 s.).

Winnicott, D. W. (1971). *Playing and reality.* London: Routledge.

Yalom, I. D. (1975). *The theory and practice of group psychotherapy.* New York: Basic Books.

CHAPTER 11

Making Meaning After Combat Trauma and Moral Injury

C.J. Button[1], J. Jinkerson[2,3], C.J. Bryan[4]
[1]United States Air Force, Little Rock Air Force Base, AR, United States; [2]Fielding Graduate University, Santa Barbara, CA, United States; [3]Air Force Institute of Technology, OH, United States; [4]The University of Utah, Salt Lake City, UT, United States

CASE VIGNETTE INTRODUCTIONS

Case Vignette #1: Sergeant First Class Robert Bicket

Sergeant First Class (SFC) Bicket presented for therapy in an undisclosed deployed location reporting impairing symptoms of guilt, shame, regret, sadness, and grief. He was physically agitated, anxious, and in significant physical pain. Through the years, he had been deployed five times in support of the US Global Wars on Terrorism. He had been hit by multiple improvised explosive devices (IEDs) and he still carried shrapnel in various locations throughout his body. He was repeatedly exposed to potentially traumatic combat events during his deployments including some of the most intense combat operations. He lost dozens of his close friends in combat and witnessed severe, life-threatening injuries to countless other Soldiers. SFC Bicket was awarded multiple Purple Hearts and was highly decorated for his valiant combat actions. He killed many enemy combatants, including some in hand-to-hand combat during his deployments. SFC Bicket's life was repeatedly threatened, and he placed himself in harm's way to safeguard other Soldiers' lives on multiple occasions.

As he retold his combat-related experiences, it became evident that he was not bothered by the grotesque minutiae of war, including all that had happened to him and all he had witnessed. He was a proud and professional Soldier who commanded deep reverence from those privileged to have met him. He was the personification of the idyllic American Soldier: the type of Soldier that little boys dreamed of becoming as they dashed about in their backyards engaging in fantasized skirmishes. He joined the military due to his deep-seeded patriotism, his ingrained belief that freedom was worth dying for, and a long family tradition of honorable military service dating back over 100 years. SFC Bicket earnestly believed in the combat mission.

Reconstructing Meaning After Trauma
ISBN 978-0-12-803015-8
http://dx.doi.org/10.1016/B978-0-12-803015-8.00011-5

He saw the benefits of the work being done each day. He understood why Coalition forces were there, and he trusted his Chain of Command. Early in his career, he dedicated himself to being the best Soldier possible and he regularly studied the tactics of great warriors who came before him. SFC Bicket was known to routinely saunter across contested battlespaces to pull inexperienced and scared Privates who were unable to muster the courage to move from the safety of their soon-to-be-compromised fighting positions, and drag them back to the safety of the squad. His men respected him—they trusted him—and they absorbed every lesson and example he furnished. Early in therapy, questions arose as to how such a brave and resilient warrior could come to suffer such impairing psychiatric symptoms.

Case Vignette #2: Staff Sergeant Ron Pash

Staff Sergeant (SSG) Pash presented for individual therapy to address symptoms of anger, anxiety, and feelings of "burn out" due to caring for veterans of his unit who were deployed to combat with him years earlier. These veterans experienced marked hardship following the war, including PTSD, depression, suicidal crises, family problems, domestic violence, substance abuse, and occupational problems. He complained of exhaustion from his tireless efforts to assist them, to keep them functioning and out of trouble, and (often) to prevent them from harming themselves. Early in their combat tour, the unit suffered heavy casualties. SSG Pash indicated that many unit members currently suffered from "survivors' guilt," blaming themselves for failing to prevent the deaths of their comrades. In fact, several wished to have died in combat alongside their friends years ago. SSG Pash denied suffering analogous tribulations. Although he too desired to thwart his friends' deaths, he acknowledged the impossible reality of the situation during the war. He recognized that he was powerless to have altered the circumstances, and he understood that he was not responsible for their deaths. His combat experiences helped him grow in an adaptive direction, as he described himself as an "asshole" before the war. Conversely, SSG Pash reported that he has since become concerned about the welfare of others, redevoted himself to his marriage, and taken great pride in raising his children. Again, questions arose early in therapy as to how someone who appeared to respond so adaptively following combat trauma could suffer psychologically all these years later.

OVERVIEW

Following life-defining experiences and highly stressful events, we are all tasked with "making meaning," or making sense, of our experiences. More so than most, our Nation's warriors must come to understand their actions and experiences in adaptive ways, or lose their well-being. For those who change during war, finding adaptive meaning is a primary force enabling them to live lives of excellence and purpose. Alternatively, maladaptive meanings forged out of one's combat experiences may lead to negative psychiatric and functional outcomes. In our clinics, we have seen our Nation's veterans reclaim their lives by going beyond correcting "irrational" thoughts. These warriors have come to understand their traumatic and worldview-jarring combat experiences in entirely new ways. They have learned to appreciate their own deeply distressing experiences through new lenses, by modifying their worldviews or reaffirming their preexisting perspectives as strong and true. In this chapter, models of meaning and meaning making following combat are presented and factors that contribute to the loss of meaning are explored. Throughout the chapter, we follow the case vignettes of SFC Bicket and SSG Pash, both of whom experienced "worldview-jarring" combat events, subsequently lost their predeployment sense of life meaning, experienced maladaptive meaning-making processes, and subsequently acquired more adaptive life meanings through therapy. The chapter concludes by addressing how the loss of meaning can be mitigated and meaning can be remade.

MEANING

In a discussion of the healing power of new meanings, it is important to understand what is meant by *meaning*. At its simplest level, meaning is a sense of purpose that contributes to a contextual framework enabling events to be interpreted (Britt, Adler, & Bartone, 2001; Bryan, Graham, & Roberge, 2015). It has to do with cognitive appraisals that are made about particular events as well as underlying self-schemas and relational schemas that filter such interpretations (Park, 2010; Slattery & Park, 2014). Meaning, however, equally has to do with the worldviews undergirding even these beliefs. From beliefs about the nature of existence and morality, to core beliefs about the self and others, to automatic attributions driven by these underlying cognitions, meaning comprises the totality of our cognitive experiences, including all beliefs that tell us what matters and what is true (Austin & Vancouver, 1996). Meaning further materializes from congruence between our value systems and our actions. That is, a life well lived is one in which our behavior is in keeping with our deeply held convictions. Such action produces a subjective sense of well-being and fullness (King, Hicks, Krull, & Del Gaiso, 2006; Park, 2010). When actions are incongruent with values, self-schemas are threatened, and resultant meaning loss takes a deep emotional toll (Baumeister, 1991; Litz et al., 2009).

In the case of warriors, meaning is often inextricably tied to the warrior ethos and core values found in each of the service branches. In combination, these tenets assert that the mission comes first and that it is executed with honor, integrity, courage, and self-sacrifice (United States Army, n.d.). In every regard, service members are to place the mission and others above themselves. Warriors believe in their ethos, which often come to dominate their global perspectives on morality. Warriors derive substantial meaning from believing that they contribute to the mission, and this imbues all of their actions with purpose.

Meaning: SFC Bicket

As to SFC Bicket's personal meaning, to say SFC Bicket was boastful would be hyperbole. He possessed a humble confidence that obligated follower-ship from those around him. He understood himself to be everything previously described and more. In short, he knew himself to be an exemplary Soldier. Service to his nation and family tradition drove him to selflessly place the combat mission and the betterment of others before himself. This was perhaps the facet of his personality that most endeared him to others. At the conclusion of his second combat tour, these beliefs, his meaning, led him to extend his combat tour. In doing so, he chose of his own volition to leave his original unit and to join a new inbound combat unit, thus enabling him to remain in theater and continue the combat mission.

Meaning: SSG Pash

Before combat, SSG Pash believed himself to be a generally good person. He loved his wife and family, but his eye would occasionally wander. At times, he "selfishly" placed his needs above those of his wife and family, and he was known to frequent local bars, come home late, and sometimes fail to fulfill promises made to his family and friends. He viewed others as being in control of their destinies, believing their circumstances were established by their actions alone (i.e., "You get what you deserve"). He generally believed himself to be a good Soldier. Before deployment, he received training focusing on the rules of engagement (ROEs) and the Law of Armed Conflict, and he believed himself to be above misconduct. Although SSG Pash did not have the immediately admirable self-sacrificial qualities of SFC Bicket, he too generally adhered to his moral principles and believed that doing so brought him sufficient karma. The days leading up to his "worldview-jarring event" were strafed with ambushes and firefights isolated to one particular neighborhood. Consequently, his unit was frustrated and tasked with going door-to-door to defeat the growing insurgency.

MEANING LOST

Because the combat theater provides increased opportunities for morally ambiguous situations, it leaves core beliefs vulnerable to meaning loss (Janoff-Bulman, 1992). As warriors experience particular emotionally and morally charged situations, they appraise these situations and make meanings for each event (Park, 2010). If situational meanings are congruent with existent beliefs, global meanings are sustained. If situational interpretations are incongruent, meaning is threatened (Park, 2010; Slattery & Park, 2014).

Meaning Lost: SFC Bicket

SFC Bicket lost meaning in the weeks following his self-determined departure from his original unit, who continued combat operations until their redeployment. His meaning was not lost through a horrifying combat experience he endured, in taking the life of an enemy combatant in a ghastly hand-to-hand struggle, or by witnessing the traumatic deaths of his fellow Soldiers. In other words, SFC Bicket did not lose meaning through a psychologically traumatic event, such as those traditionally associated with PTSD. After leaving his original unit, SFC Bicket's original team (absent SFC Bicket) came under enemy fire. During the operation, the new team leader gave a lawful order, which ran contrary to SFC Bicket's personal standard operating procedures. While following that order, three of SFC Bicket's former teammates came under heavy fire and died by multiple gunshot wounds. Following their deaths, SFC Bicket concluded that his men—his friends—died because he "selfishly" extended his combat tour. He believed that if he had been on patrol with his Soldiers that day, they would have lived. He was convinced that he would have performed better on the battlefield that day. He was certain that had he remained with his original unit, he would have made an alternate and better order, thereby preventing their deaths, as the team would not have been overpowered. He even went so far as to state that because he was fighting strongly in another part of the theater with his new unit, he likely pushed additional enemy forces in the direction of his former unit, thus ensuring their inevitable deaths.

Meaning Lost: SSG Pash

For SSG Pash, meaning was lost following days of ambushes, firefights, and the ensuing combat injuries that inescapably result. On the day he felt his meaning was lost, SSG Pash's unit was tasked with going door-to-door in the neighborhood where the ambushes were centered. After hours of frustrating and life-threatening work, his unit entered the home of a local man and his wife, where they unearthed a cache of firearms and ammunition. In essence, his unit found the epicenter of the insurgency's supply lines. During questioning, the local man became argumentative, aggressive, and lunged at SSG Pash. In response, SSG Pash subdued the man by punching him in the face, drawing his firearm on the man, and threatening to use it if the man failed to comply. After arresting the man, his wife became similarly argumentative and physically aggressive toward SSG Pash. After multiple attempts to verbally calm her, she too hurled herself at SSG Pash intending to assault him and likely cause bodily harm. Instinctively, SSG Pash reacted in an analogous manner to subdue the local woman. He landed a crushing blow to her forehead, thrusting her backward, where she landed in a heap. She also happened to be pregnant, which SSG Pash knew before striking her.

MALADAPTIVE AND ADAPTIVE MEANING

Traumatic Maladaptive Meaning

Many warriors experience the combat deaths of their comrades analogous to those reported by SFC Bicket. That is, as much as they refuse to accept this reality, warriors are unable to prevent the combat deaths of their comrades. Many warriors also tend to hold a just world belief, such that combat death only occurs to morally deserving individuals (Janoff-Bulman, 1992). This belief is one factor, along with many others, that aids in overcoming our shared and innate psychological reluctance to kill other humans. When their comrades die, however, warriors who hold the just world belief are confronted with incompatible information: their comrades, whom they believed to be good people and thereby deserving of good outcomes, have been killed. Warriors are then faced with at least two options for alleviating cognitive dissonance: maintain the just world belief, thereby requiring acceptance that comrades "earned" their deaths through some moral deficiencies, or abandon the just world belief and subsequently threaten core beliefs about causation, morality, and locus of control.

Traumatic Adaptive Meaning

Yet another option for warriors is to change, or accommodate, global belief to become more flexible and adaptive in light of life experiences. In doing so, warriors engage in the meaning making process, which involves searching for a way to (1) understand the situation and/or (2) attribute significance or assign meaning to it. For instance, a single warrior may adopt the reasonable perspective that, "Terrible things happen in life, and there is sometimes no good explanation for why these terrible things occur." Should a warrior adopt this viewpoint, he will likely be subjectively absolved of the guilt associated with "failing" to prevent one's comrades' deaths. Such a conclusion, however, does not satisfy the emotional weight of losing one's friends and blaming oneself. Emotional processing is needed in addition to cognitive processing. Through these dual processes, the warrior may indeed come to recognize that he does not bear guilt. This experience may, however, require a spiritual change and/or shift in identity (Park, 2010).

Maladaptive Meaning and Moral Injury

Warrior science has begun to recognize a particular type of trauma associated with the dissonance of acting incongruently with one's personal values (Litz et al., 2009). This moral injury is characterized by intense guilt and shame, spiritual/existential crisis, loss of trust in self, and loss of subjective meaning in life. It is likewise associated with a host of psychiatric problems including depression, anxiety, reexperiencing, self-punishment/self-harm, and suicidal ideation, as well as social problems (Drescher et al., 2011; Jinkerson, in preparation). Models of moral injury (Litz et al., 2009) easily align with the general meaning making model (Park, 2010), such that moral injury can be construed as a syndrome of lost meanings.

According to Litz et al. (2009) moral injury model, when one's actions are demonstrably inconsistent with his/her personal moral values, it creates moral dissonance. Examples include killing in combat, but are often more closely related to combat actions that result in the killing of individuals traditionally defined as noncombatants (i.e., particularly women, the elderly, and children as commonly occurs in asymmetric warfare), even when these individuals are engaged in actions that clearly identify them as enemy combatants (Vargas, Hanson, Kraus, Drescher, & Foy, 2013). Moral dissonance may be resolved through appropriate assimilation or accommodation. For instance, a warrior may believe that killing civilians is wrong. However, while adhering to the ROEs, he may ultimately find that he must kill an individual (who initially used his/her gender or age to conceal himself/herself as a noncombatant so as to gain a tactical advantage) to protect his comrades and the mission. If he is able to quickly resolve this conflict by recognizing his adherence to overall moral principles (i.e., protection, ROEs, just war), this cognitive accommodation avoids psychological damage. If, on the other hand, the warrior is unable to rectify the disparity between his/her lawful combat actions and his personal moral values (e.g., "thou shalt not kill," particularly women, children, and the elderly), shame and guilt will invariably result. Within the warrior's spiritual world, he comes to believe he is damaged and evil, so he erroneously condemns himself and refuses forgiveness. Due to believing himself morally stained, he may engage in self-harm, self-handicapping, avoidance of memories, and numbing himself to emotion (Litz et al., 2009).

In the aforementioned example, moral injury develops through situational attribution, which is itself interpreted through global beliefs such as "I'm a good person." When one acts inconsistently with his personal morals/beliefs and cannot rectify the disparity, it is not possible to maintain a positive self-concept or a fulfilling relationship with a higher power. Meaning lost through moral injury includes self-identity, subjective purpose, and metaphysical connection, whereas the meaning made following moral injury is one of the self as broken, sinful, damaged, and beyond redemption.

Although moral injury shares some symptoms with PTSD (e.g., both conditions develop after intensely stressful situations and they frequently co-occur), there are several important distinctions (Hendin & Haas, 1991; Resick, Monson, & Chard, 2014, pp. 73–78). Moral injury develops through a failure to resolve the moral dissonance between one's actions and personal values, whereas PTSD develops through exposure to a traumatic (i.e., psychologically and life-threatening) event. Because the combat theater (particularly one ripe with asymmetric warfare) provides a backdrop wherein decisions (with moral underpinnings) are made and life is threatened routinely, it is not surprising that the same events may produce both moral injury and PTSD (Hendin & Haas, 1991; Mental Health Advisory Team, 2008). Moreover, because moral injuries may lead to the development of more significant psychiatric symptoms, moral injury may be a precursor to protracted PTSD presentations. Specifically, negative global beliefs that develop on the battlefield, such as "I'm a monster" or "God hates me," along with associated guilt and shame (i.e., moral injury) are often the complicating factors interfering with posttraumatic stress recovery (Riggs, Rothbaum,

& Foa, 1995). As a result, identifying factors that facilitate and contribute to meaning change in combat may help mitigate the development of moral injury as well as PTSD.

Maladaptive Meaning: SFC Bicket

As to the maladaptive meanings that SFC Bicket developed, he stated, "I am a total disappointment. I failed as a Soldier and as a leader. I might as well have been the one to pull the trigger. My selfish decision killed them all!" SFC Bicket exclaimed that his decision to leave his original unit directly resulted in the deaths of three of his former team members. He blamed himself for leaving them vulnerable with what he believed was a poor leader and a poor warfighter, whom they naïvely followed to their deaths. He wholeheartedly believed that had he been present on the battlefield that day, his friends would still be alive. SFC Bicket continued, "I have betrayed everything I believe in…my country, the Army, my family…and most importantly, all my Soldiers…all of them that I have ever led. I have dishonored everyone who has come before me."

Maladaptive Meaning: SSG Pash

After subduing the local woman, SSG Pash initially saw no wrong in his actions. However, he began to waver just moments after the incident and questioned himself, "What the hell am I doing? Have I slumped so low that I believe it is okay to punch a pregnant woman?" Those words deeply troubled SSG Pash and they echoed in his mind for weeks following the event. His actions ran contrary to everything he had been taught and believed. "You never hit women! How could I have done that? What the hell is wrong with me?" he emphatically proclaimed years later in therapy.

Several weeks after the incident involving the pregnant local woman, SSG Pash's unit suffered heavy casualties in an IED ambush that took several Soldiers' lives. Years later in therapy, SSG Pash found himself still haunted by his questions. He explained that after he punched the woman, he noticed a blood stain quickly forming on her clothing and running downward as she struggled to gather herself and slowly staggered to stand up. He stated that she fled to her neighbors' home to tend to her injury. SSG Pash never saw her again. He concluded that after he struck the woman and she collapsed to the floor, she had miscarried her unborn child, hence the blood he had observed. Following the event, he was convinced that word spread throughout the neighborhood of the harm an American Soldier had brought upon this woman and her unborn child. As a result, he believed that locals, still undecided regarding the American presence, joined the insurgency. In doing so, these new insurgents, borne out of his misconduct, sought to avenge the death of this unborn child. In an act of revenge, he believed that they planted the IED and launched the ambush on his unit that killed his friends weeks after he struck the woman. In his words, "I am a horrible person. It's entirely my fault. I killed them all. This never would have happened if it weren't for me. What I did was reprehensible. I am to blame."

FACTORS AFFECTING MEANING MAKING AND LOSS

Although most combatants experience potentially morally injurious events, few develop moral injury. Differences between those who suffer moral injury and those who resolve moral conflict is not readily understood, but it has been proposed that stable, internal attributions moderate moral injury's development (Litz et al., 2009). That is, holding specific existing meanings and meaning combinations may protect combatants from meaning loss and moral injury. Such protective meaning may come from worldview, personal morals/ethics, spiritual beliefs, global beliefs (i.e., self- and relational schemas), and subjective meaning in life.

Collectively, these factors represent a cognitive topography such that each factor informs the next, and each level contributes to overall meaning and psychological health (Jinkerson, in preparation; Koltko-Rivera, 2004). Worldview represents individuals' fundamental beliefs about the universe, including issues of what exists, human nature, values, and how one relates to existence (Jinkerson, in preparation; Kolto-Rivera, 2004). As it relates to meanings carried into and taken from combat, worldview provides a basis upon which spiritual significance may be built. For instance, one must believe that human nature is malleable before one can accept forgiveness. Global beliefs are also built upon worldview. The just world belief, for example, is more likely to be found among spiritualists than materialists. Emergent from these three levels is subjective meaning in life. One's worldview, spiritual beliefs, and beliefs about the self/others contribute to one's understanding of what matters. Pursuit of, and congruence with, one's personal mattering builds personal fulfillment. In the case of our Nation's warriors, when the just world belief is combined with the warrior ethos, little room is left for ambiguity.

On existing models of moral injury, two things make moral injury (i.e., meanings lost) more likely. First, having underdeveloped internal attributions makes moral conflict more likely. That is, individuals with less defined worldviews, less understood and integrated spiritual understanding, poorly defined and developed morals, and/or unsupported global beliefs are much more likely to encounter moral conflict (Harris, Park, Currier, Usset, & Voecks, 2015; Jinkerson, in preparation). This is because their internal cognitive structures have not been reinforced with reality congruence. The second is that rigid beliefs are more likely to contribute to moral injury. When one's global beliefs are filled with nuance, recognition of variable moral application, and an acknowledgment that one's existing knowledge base is incomplete, it is more difficult to shake one's cognitive foundation (Park, 2010; Slattery & Park, 2014).

Factors Affecting SFC Bicket

In SFC Bicket's case, his worldview included believing that the Chain of Command is sacred, actions ought to be performed for the good of the group, humans are free moral agents, each person is responsible for his own outcomes, human nature is modifiable, and there is an objective moral set. His values epistemology was deeply rooted in the warrior ethos and Army core values. For SFC Bicket, the spiritual significance of sacrifice, or the meaning of a warrior's death, emerged from actions taken consistent with the warrior ethos. Namely, SFC Bicket reasoned that he violated the central tenets of that ethos by "selfishly" extending his combat tour, or in his mind, abandoning his brothers-in-arms. This was in turn a perceived violation of the principle of self-sacrifice, the moral and professional value that SFC Bicket cherished above all others. This perceived violation was equally a destruction of SFC Bicket's reverence of the Chain of Command and collectivistic beliefs. Since SFC Bicket recognized his actions as voluntary and held himself responsible for life's successes and failures, he believed that his actions had grievance consequences. He had, in essence, stripped his friends' sacrifice of nobility, leaving their loss utterly meaningless.

Factors Affecting SSG Pash

SSG Pash's worldview and moral understanding were not particularly developed. He believed in some objective values but viewed moral duties as fluid. He generally valued the Chain of Command and adherence to the ROEs, but he sometimes acted in selfish ways. Because SSG Pash did not have a strong moral epistemology and had insufficiently internalized the Army's core values, it is no surprise that he did not initially experience a moral conflict. Only upon later reflection that his actions were (outside of their actual context) morally abhorrent did he consider how he was living. SSG

Pash also appears to have held the just world belief. That belief was shaken when he found himself acting in a manner that he never believed he would. According to the just world perspective, either the woman deserved what she got or he would soon be punished by his actions. Consequently, SSG Pash more thoroughly embraced the warrior ethos from that point forward, became more self-sacrificial, and adopted a collectivistic perspective toward others. His just world belief, however, remained rigid, as he attempted to repair the perceived damage done to his karma through action rather than engage in noble pursuits as means unto themselves.

CLINICAL IMPLICATIONS

As SFC Bicket's and SSG Pash's stories demonstrate, these are tales not just of becoming broken but also of being made whole. In some ways, therapies in common practice [e.g., Cognitive Processing Therapy (CPT), Cognitive Therapy, Acceptance and Commitment Therapy, and Existential Therapy] are already prepared to address the meanings lost and the moral dissonance that emerge from combat.

In particular, CPT asserts that negative shifts in global beliefs complicate traumatic recovery. In response, CPT recommends that negatively modified cognitions be addressed directly so that more flexible cognitive alternatives may be adopted (Resick et al., 2014, pp. 3, 31–36, and 95–124). In the case of SFC Bicket, who failed to prevent others' deaths, he believed that he should have stopped their deaths somehow, so he felt morally responsible for their loss of life. CPT can assist in such cases by acknowledging the limited options that were available in the moment, which can be very powerful in decreasing guilt. Such cognitive restructuring strategies are often possible even when self-schemas have been damaged.

Sometimes, worldview itself may need to be modified. For instance, if an individual with moral injury believes himself to be evil and that he cannot change his nature, it is necessary to help him recognize that humans can change. This may be done with competitive evidence, but it may be more effective to work within the person's spiritual framework to identify religious, spiritual, or humanistic beliefs that allow for forgiveness or a values-driven life. Similarly, if a warrior believes that he has committed a serious moral violation, it may be possible to help him broaden his ethical perspective within his own religious or spiritual framework. In some instances, individuals truly have done terrible things. When they acknowledge the possibility of forgiveness, it is possible to approach forgiveness through religious and/or spiritual rites, including atonement, penitence, confession, prayer/mediation, and self-compassion (Cukor, Spitalnick, Difede, Rizzo, & Rothbaum, 2009). Through this holistic integration of mind and spirit, a subjective sense of meaning often reemerges (Harris et al., 2011; Litz et al., 2009). Because additional emotional processing and working through is needed to reachieve meaning and personal purpose, correcting irrational thoughts alone is often insufficient (Park, 2010).

Remaking meaning is not always best suited for the clinic, however. Meaning is achieved within personal cultures, religious spheres, and local communities. Because meanings lost may lead to depression and withdrawal, healing these losses requires reintegration of affected individuals into their peer groups. It may require peer mentoring, competing information from moral authorities, or communal story sharing (Buechner, 2014; Cukor et al., 2009). In the community setting, the healing functions are essentially the same as the clinic, but warriors' existence outside of a pathologizing environment and surrounded by supportive friends may naturally alleviate shame. Likewise, peers and spiritual authorities can assist in identifying possible meanings of stressful experiences. When stories of meanings lost are shared with others, new communal meanings may emerge, which provide a comforting sense of truth and perspective (Buechner, 2014).

Meaning Remade: SFC Bicket

SFC Bicket presented to therapy nearly 7 years after his friends' deaths. He was initially slow to reveal the extent of his psychiatric concerns. His maladaptive meaning was well guarded, and he hid behind anger, fantastically incredible stories of war, and a prideful façade of excitement as he recounted his combat actions. Although he did not explicitly define his preexisting meaning, it nonetheless emerged insidiously as therapy progressed. As rapport continued to strengthen, his defenses gradually lowered, and he revealed the full extent of his guilt, shame, and maladaptive meaning.

Over the course of therapy, little by little, he began to appreciate the fact that he was there on the battlefield alongside his men on the day they died. He understood he was not there physically, but in terms of the wisdom he had imparted upon his men and the character he had developed in them. Again, he blamed himself for their deaths because he believed they had been provided a poor leader in his absence, whom they naïvely followed to their deaths. He believed that he hand delivered that leader to them when he decided to "selfishly" leave them to extend his combat tour. When he was able to work through the event resulting in their deaths, he acknowledged several new perspectives. He appreciated the limits of his initial perspective, as he viewed that leader through hindsight and knew full well the outcome of his decision that day. More importantly, he discovered that his men had acted courageously and selflessly. He understood that his Soldiers—his friends—had acted with no greater love: that they had laid down their lives so that others may live. He had failed to remember where and how they were found. Their bodies were discovered on the battlefield, offset and alongside one another. Their weapons were drawn and pointing down range and on target. According to SFC Bicket, they were found in "textbook assault formation," and yet not a single bullet had been discharged from their weapons.

In recounting the details of the event, SFC Bicket came to realize that they had willfully withheld fire upon enemy combatants who were using noncombatants—women and children—as human shields, a fact he had long since dismissed as irrelevant. These selfless and brave American Soldiers knowingly and selflessly chose their own deaths over risking the lives of innocent women and children intentionally placed in harm's way by the enemy. His Soldiers followed his example and the guidance he had always furnished to them. He came to believe that he was there with them on that day. He realized that they could have selfishly fought for their lives and risked the lives of those innocent women and children, but instead they all selflessly and freely chose their deaths. He understood that there was nothing he could have done to have prevented their deaths. In remaking meaning, he understood that he had adequately prepared them to act with nobility and courage. He shifted his view of his men from one of naïveté to one of heroism. In making this new meaning, he was able to release his guilt. He also acknowledged his selflessness and the countless lives saved by his continued and positive presence during the 11 months that followed their deaths while completing his extended combat tour.

Meaning Remade: SSG Pash

Therapy initially focused on helping SSG Pash set boundaries and relinquish responsibility for the current well-being of his former unit members. Although he was less stressed, he realized little symptomatic relief as he let go of his current responsibility for others' emotions and conduct. Therapeutic progress was initially sluggish, and SSG Pash regularly failed to attend his appointments. In his ninth session, he finally revealed the nature of his concerns involving the local woman. In the sessions that followed, he relayed how he believed his actions culminated in the combat injuries and deaths of several unit members.

In the decade since the ambush, he described how he sought to atone for what he had done and all that he believed he had caused. He introspectively questioned who he was before the war, and he determined to lay aside his selfish pride and instead seek humility, atonement, individual growth, and the betterment of those around him. He acknowledged that he was an "asshole" before the war and he resolved to rectify his prewar shortcomings. He devoted himself to being present and active in the lives of his wife and children, and he found new meaning in fatherhood. He renewed his religious and spiritual beliefs and routinely volunteered to aid those less fortunate than himself. He devoted himself to caring for unit members who bore the physical and psychological injuries of war. In essence, he had become a new man, a changed man, and a better man than he was before the war.

Yet, despite all the altruistic endeavors and the positive changes he made personally, he found no solace, no respite, no resolution to the shame and guilt he bore for having struck the pregnant woman. Through therapy, he studied the event in infinite detail. Every facet of his memory was examined and Socratically confronted. What emerged was an entirely different conclusion. He came to believe that his punch could not have caused a miscarriage. He acknowledged that the womb is highly protective. He remembered that the woman landed on her backside and that at no point did her belly come into contact with a hard surface. He recalled that she was wearing black clothing and therefore, he could not have discerned blood from urine. Further, he acknowledged that blood does not flow or absorb into fabric as quickly as he had observed. Rather, what he observed was more consistent with urine.

He concluded that she likely lost control of her bladder due to her pregnancy and/or a sympathetic nervous system-related fear response, as she had only moments earlier witnessed her husband's life threatened after he had engaged in similar combative behavior. In retrospect, he determined that she likely had not miscarried. As a result, he acknowledged that his misconduct most likely had not brought about the development of new insurgents. Therefore, the ambush that caused the injuries and deaths of many of his unit members was not attributable to his actions. Rather, the ambush was a natural consequence of war and not borne out of his actions.

Although he continued to regret having struck the woman, he acknowledged, "Ironically, it was probably one of the best things that ever happened in my life." He continued, "Therapy is bittersweet...I find it rewarding and frustrating. Today I realized that I have wasted the last decade atoning for an

IED that I didn't cause. It seems so obvious looking at it now. Yet, I know that had I not viewed it in that manner, I would probably still be the same asshole I was ten years ago. I know I am a better person today because of what I did. I wish I could ask her for her forgiveness, what I did was inexcusable. Sadly, hitting her was my impetus for change. I still have a ways to go; life is about continually growing as a person. I just hope next time I need an impetus, I don't have to do something regretful to realize I need to change as a person. I think she would find some peace in knowing that this has changed me for the better." Even in his final reflections, he still was not able to fully release the negative characterization of his actions that day, which were completely appropriate in the context of the burgeoning assaultive situation. Indeed, one additional meaning SSG Pash might have made is that his actions (i.e., deescalating a hostile situation using the minimum necessary amount of force) likely avoided any Coalition casualties and kept the woman and her husband from becoming further and more seriously harmed.

CONCLUDING REMARKS

If we help our Nation's warriors reclaim meaning in life, we accept a worthwhile burden as well. Years of PTSD research and misunderstandings about the wounds of war sometimes cloud our perspectives and leave us believing that warriors sacrifice only to return broken and unhealed. Most warriors, however, derive great meaning from their service to country, and it is the rest of us who must come to better understand their purpose and perspective. As providers, we can seek to better understand the cognitive and emotional factors contributing to meanings lost in combat, and we can Socratically assist our warriors in recognizing errors in their cognition. This is indeed a healing process. Without community integration, spiritual understanding, and the mutual feeling that psychotherapy is rooted in, however, we cannot hope for that to be enough. What is enough is for us to enter into the warrior ethos ourselves, to embrace the perspective that change is possible, and to believe that in helping our warriors find meaning in life, we may find our own. Often, as these two case vignettes illustrate, the invisible wounds of war are cautiously revealed through the safety and trust of a nonjudgmental, patient, and empathic therapeutic relationship. In each case, the true nature of their distress was not revealed until 9 or 10 sessions into treatment. Clinicians are encouraged to be patient with our combat veterans, particularly if treatment seems to be slow or stalled. In the case of moral injury, it appears they clearly seek a strong and trusting therapeutic alliance before disclosing the full extent of their concerns.

The work we do is powerful and meaningful change can come about quickly once these maladaptive meanings are revealed and targeted in therapy.

In his final words before termination, SFC Bicket reminds us of the importance of our work as he stated, "Combat was my life, killing and destroying my way through the last 10 years. I cannot express how grateful I really am for all you have done. You really are amazing. I will always remember my work with you. For the very short time we spent talking about all of it…it truly changed my life and allowed me to fully honor the service, sacrifice, and spirit of my friends. Thanks again Doc! Thanks for helping me find my meaning and purpose once more. I hope my story helps others to heal!"

AUTHORS' NOTE

The names of the Soldiers depicted in the case vignettes are pseudonyms. All personally identifying information has been altered to protect their identities. The Soldiers' combat experiences and clinical disclosures have been modified to further obscure identification, while still maintaining the fidelity of their stories. Thus, any similarities between the Soldiers depicted in these case vignettes and any individuals known to the reader are purely coincidental and likely represent the ubiquitous nature of their experiences. The Soldiers depicted provided voluntary signed written informed consent agreeing to the use of their deidentified and modified stories for use in this chapter.

DISCLAIMER

The views expressed in this chapter are those of the authors and do not necessarily reflect the official policy or position of the US Government, the Department of Defense, the Department of the Air Force, or the Department of the Army.

REFERENCES

Austin, J. T., & Vancouver, J. B. (1996). Goal constructs in psychology: structure, process, and content. *Psychological Bulletin, 120*, 338–375.

Baumeister, R. (1991). *Meanings of life.* New York, NY: Guilford Press.

Britt, T. W., Adler, A. B., & Bartone, P. T. (2001). Deriving benefits from stressful events: the role of engagement in meaningful work and hardiness. *Journal of Occupational Health Psychology, 1*, 56–63.

Bryan, C. J., Graham, E., & Roberge, E. (2015). Living a life worth living: spirituality and suicide risk in military personnel. *Spirituality in Clinical Practice, 2*(1), 74–78.

Buechner, B. D. (2014). *Contextual mentoring of student veterans: A communication perspective* (Doctoral dissertation). Santa Barbara, CA: Fielding Graduate University.

Cukor, J., Spitalnick, J., Difede, J., Rizzo, A. A., & Rothbaum, B. O. (2009). Emerging treatments for PTSD. *Clinical Psychology Review, 29*(8), 715–726.

Drescher, K., Foy, D., Litz, B. T., Kelly, C., Leshner, A., & Schultz, K. (2011). An exploration of the viability and usefulness of the construct of moral injury in war veterans. *Traumatology, 17*, 8–13. http://dx.doi.org/10.1177/1534765610395615.

Harris, J. I., Erbes, C. R., Engdahl, B. E., Thuras, P., Murray-Swank, N., ... & Le, T. (2011). *The effectiveness of a trauma-focused spiritually integrated intervention for veterans exposed to trauma.*

Harris, J. I., Park, C. L., Currier, J. M., Usset, T. J., & Voecks, C. D. (2015). Moral injury and psycho-spiritual development: considering the developmental context. *Spirituality in Clinical Practice, 2.* http://dx.doi.org/10.1037/scp0000045 (Online early publication).

Hendin, H., & Haas, A. P. (1991). Suicide and guilt as manifestations of PTSD in Vietnam combat veterans. *American Journal of Psychiatry, 148*(5), 586–591.

Janoff-Bulman, R. (1992). *Shattered assumptions: Towards a new psychology of trauma.* New York, NY: Free Press.

Jinkerson, J.D. (in preparation). Moral injury in combat veterans: A theoretical and empirical explanation of the moderating role of worldview relationships.

King, L. A., Hicks, J. A., Krull, J. L., & Del Gaiso, A. K. (2006). Positive affect and the experience of meaning in life. *Journal of Personality and Social Psychology, 90*, 179–196.

Koltko-Rivera, M. E. (2004). The psychology of worldviews. *Review of General Psychology, 8*(1), 3–58.

Litz, B. T., Stein, N., Delaney, E., Lebowitz, L., Nash, W. P., Silva, C., & Maguen, S. (2009). Moral injury and moral repair in war veterans: a preliminary model and intervention strategy. *Clinical Psychology Review, 29*(8), 695–706.

Mental Health Advisory Team. (2008). *MHAT-V 2008 report.* Retrieved from http://army-medicine.mil/Documents/Redacted1-MHATV-4-FEB-2008-Overview.pdf.

Park, C. L. (2010). Making sense of the meaning literature: an integrative review of meaning making and its effects on adjustment to stressful life events. *Psychological Bulletin, 136*, 257–301. http://dx.doi.org/10.1037/a0018301.

Resick, P. A., Monson, C. M., & Chard, K. M. (2014). *Cognitive processing therapy: Veteran/military version: Therapist's manual.* Washington, DC: Department of Veteran Affairs.

Riggs, D. S., Rothbaum, B. O., & Foa, E. B. (1995). A prospective examination of symptoms of posttraumatic stress disorder in victims of nonsexual assault. *Journal of Interpersonal Violence, 10*(2), 201–204.

Slattery, J. M., & Park, C. L. (2014). Spirituality and meaning making: implications for therapy with trauma survivors. In D. F. Wlker, C. A. Courtois, & J. D. Aten (Eds.), *Spiritually oriented psychotherapy for trauma* (pp. 127–146). Washington, DC: APA.

United States Army, (n.d.). *The Army values.* Retrieved from http://www.army.mil/values/.

Vargas, A. F., Hanson, T., Kraus, D., Drescher, K., & Foy, D. (2013). Moral injury themes in combat veterans' narrative responses from the national Vietnam veterans' readjustment study. *Traumatology, 19*(3), 243–250.

PART 4

Conclusion

CHAPTER 12

Meaning Making and Trauma Recovery

C.A. Courtois
Independent Practice, (retired), Washington, DC, United States

Trauma, by its very nature, destroys absolutes: it causes interruption and discontinuity as it shatters life as it was lived and understood. It is often a marker of what was before and what was after, not only concerning circumstance and context (e.g., before the war, rape, tornado, or accident) but also in terms of the victim's sense of self (e.g., many survivors describe selves that are distinctly bifurcated into "before" and "after"). In fact, this is so normative that Van der Hart, Nijenhuis, and Steele (2006) in their study of trauma describe a posttraumatic split self. It consists of an "apparently normal" personality (ANP) that goes on with normal life activities, separated from the emotional or traumatized personality (EP), all in a valiant attempt to get over and not remember or reexperience the trauma and to leave it behind. The very nature and definition of trauma make it different than what most consider normal life (although we now know that far too many unfortunate individuals and communities are suffused in ongoing and cumulative experiences of trauma that constitute what normal is for them) (Kira, 2010). Whether in the aftermath of one-time or time-limited trauma or in the midst of continuous trauma, victims (and their loved ones and other caregivers) are left to deal with its reality and to make sense of it, even when there is no sense to be made and no logic or rhyme or reason to explain what occurred or why.

The chapters of this book provide testament to the many diverse ways that trauma can impact individuals, communities, and societies and the many interpretations and meanings that are possible. The chapters illustrate that not all individuals (and communities and societies, for that matter) respond in the same way even if they experienced the same traumatic circumstance. There are highly subjective and idiosyncratic dimensions to victims' responses. These can impede resolution and lead to posttraumatic decline (up to and including poor health and early death and suicide) or can resolve in a way that results in posttraumatic growth and positive transformation. Some

Reconstructing Meaning After Trauma
ISBN 978-0-12-803015-8
http://dx.doi.org/10.1016/B978-0-12-803015-8.00012-7

victims/survivors are more resilient than others and it takes much more to impact them. In these chapters, we learn about the process of meaning making and recovery and the various ways that these can come about. The challenge for the therapist is to deeply understand how each individual client comprehends the traumatization and how he or she ascribes meaning to it. Through this process, the therapist hopefully finds ways to influence this meaning in the direction of resolution in order for traumatic memories and emotions to become more like those of normal life events and to no longer hijack the victim's physiology and psychology.

Wilson (1989) provided a theoretical Person × Environment (P × E) model that is very helpful to therapists and their clients as they attempt to make sense and meaning of what happened to them. This model is highly compatible with the philosophical foundations of the specialization of counseling psychology with its focus on normative development and the individual's subjectivity (person) in interaction with context (environment). It suggests that the individual must be understood personally, as concerns his or her unique and idiosyncratic self (temperament, developmental history, family background and attachment style, gender, and culture, among other diversity and contextual factors), objectively, as concerns the specifics of the traumatic occurrence to gain information about what might have been most shocking and disturbing to the victim, and subjectively, in terms of the how he or she experienced it and made sense of it at the time and in its aftermath.

The contemporary study of trauma has deepened understanding of the trauma response and outcomes and, in the process, has found support for Wilson's model and for the subjective nature of an individual's response. For example, it should not be assumed that all trauma results in the development of posttraumatic stress disorder (PTSD). Research data have been consolidated to suggest that the majority of adults who are traumatized in some major way have normative posttraumatic reactions that, once faced and processed (i.e., not actively avoided or not split off into the ANP and EP selves described by Van der Hart et al., 2006 and discussed earlier), do not develop into symptoms that meet criteria for the diagnosis of PTSD (Yehuda, 1999). Rather, approximately one-third of traumatized adults go on to develop PTSD and two-thirds do not. Some develop symptoms of acute stress response that resolve within a month of the trauma. There are some exceptions to these findings in that risk factors for greater severity of response have been identified (including gender, age and maturity, duration and severity of trauma, and relationship between perpetrator and victim) and some types of trauma (notably, rape and combat, continuous and cumulative trauma). In contrast, children have higher risk for PTSD due to their dependency and physical and psychological immaturity. They have much less capacity to understand and process their reactions alone without the support, reassurance, and explanation of their caretakers. Although dissociation occurs quite routinely in response to adult-onset trauma, it is especially likely to occur in children who are more developmentally primed to dissociate, especially when the traumatic circumstances are ongoing and when there is no escape and no source of solace or support (Putnam, 1997).

Research findings from the neurosciences are providing another dimension to the P × E equation, namely, the victim's physiological response at the time of the trauma and afterward. The danger associated with the traumatization activates the individual's stress response and defensive reactions. Fight or flight is the initial autonomic impulse, based on the activation of the amygdala and other parts of the limbic system and messages from the central nervous system. This response is one of hyperarousal of the physiology. When the danger is prolonged, however, or when other risk factors are present, the response can become one of hypoarousal involving physical collapse and tonic immobility. Individuals who develop PTSD often alternate between reexperiencing accompanied by physiological activation and hypervigilance (hyperarousal) and numbing, forgetting, and depersonalization/derealization/dissociation (hypoarousal). In active PTSD, the physiology and psychology are "stuck," caught between over- and underarousal in response to reminders of the trauma (commonly referred to as triggers). As long as the trauma is not faced or resolved in some way and as long as the ANP and the EP remain split, the response is likely to continue, causing the individual to remain symptomatic and to be "hijacked" by PTSD symptoms when they encounter a traumatic reminder. When the split is identified and approached rather than avoided, the potential for change opens up.

The psychology of the trauma response is certainly affected by the physiology of PTSD but the response is a reciprocal one. This is accounted for in the expanded diagnostic criteria of PTSD in the newly revised *Diagnostic and Statistical Manual of Mental Disorders (DSM)*, Fifth Edition (American Psychiatric Association, 2013) now characterized by four core symptom clusters (1) recurrent, involuntary, and intrusive recollections of the event; (2) avoidance of stimuli associated with the trauma; (3) negative alterations in cognitions or moods associated with the event, or numbing (or both); and (4) alterations in arousal and reactivity, including a heightened sensitivity to potential threat, as opposed to three symptom clusters

(1) reexperiencing, (2) avoidance and numbing, and (3) hyperarousal contained in the previous version, *DSM*, Fourth Edition, Text Revision (American Psychiatric Association, 2000). This new diagnostic formulation accounts for the alternating arousal patterns but goes beyond them and gives more specificity to another response dimension, that of negative subjective changes in the individual in terms of beliefs and cognitions associated with worldview/spirituality, self-esteem, and relations with others. These include many of the meaning-making issues, "stuck points," and personal resilience discussed in the chapters of this book.

Put another way, the psychological response to trauma follows the physiological in the sense that responses can get stuck in one pole or the other in a way that does not allow them to be processed or integrated. Like physiological responses of overreactivity on the one hand or underreactivity/ numbness on the other, psychological responses tend to rigidify if left unrecognized and unaddressed, making the individual vulnerable in a different way to reminders of the trauma that trigger the posttraumatic response. What this suggests, and what is so well represented in the chapters of this book, is the necessity to help the client to move from a position of irresolution (and possibly even entrenchment) to one that is more worked out and settled. It implies a process that is dynamic rather than static and thus is what opens up the possibility for change and healing.

RECOVERY AND RESTORATION

So how does a victim come to terms with horrendous events and experiences and the terrible knowledge (Jay, 1991) that accompanies these? How does a victim achieve some degree of resolution or forgiveness, make meaning, or make peace with God, self, perpetrators, and others? I suggest it is not only the processing of the symptoms of the trauma itself (as implied by many trauma-focused treatments, some of which do have a cognitive processing or meaning-making component) but also the context of the treatment and the relationship with the psychotherapist and/or with others who have gone through similar experiences. As noted by Altmaier (2016) in her introductory chapter, healing occurs in the context of safety, trustworthiness, respect, collaboration, empowerment, and the support of others, that is, through connection and reconnection.

Understandably, interpersonal trauma, especially when it involves a high degree of betrayal, creates heightened mistrust of self and others (Freyd, 1998). Lifson (1979) described trauma as a "break in the human lifeline." A restoration of the lifeline through connection with caring and attuned others offers hope and a way out. A context of safety and security must be created and the psychotherapist and others must have the capacity to listen deeply and to understand and respect the uniqueness of the individual, while remaining emotionally regulated in response. As described earlier, experiences of trauma and responses to it vary dramatically. It is up to the therapist to assist clients in identifying their own distinctive responses and through the provision of information, and intense and directed discussion in the context of support/connection to help them come to terms with what happened to them and to move beyond their stuck points. It is also helpful that the therapist not hold specific expectations of meaning making or of healing for the client and instead to expect that each one will heal at his or her own pace and in dramatically different ways. Methods of healing and the meaning of resolution are enormously diverse.

Altmaier (2016) began this book by discussing the definition of recovery and posited it as more than the absence of negatives or the presence of positives. It is active rather than passive or static, as indicated by her statement that "This book is predicated on the notion that meaning is a *movement* from a word or group of words to an interpretation" (p. xv). She also noted that recovery and its associated meaning making often involve great struggle and effort on the part of the individual or the community and may be impacted by cultural factors or other belief systems. Like other processes of change, recovery is not linear, and may occur in fits and starts, and in trial and error. It may need to be "tried on." As suggested in the second and third sections of this book, it also is determined by the victim's identity and context and by the type of trauma experienced.

Recovery and restoration are words that begin with the prefix "re-." So do other related terms such as *re*demption, *re*silience, *re*stitution, *re*newal, *re*solution, *re*working, and *re*conciliation, among many others. I am indebted to psychologist Donald Meichenbaum for raising my awareness of the significance of this prefix. It generally connotes a return to a previous condition, a *re*petition, or *re*storation. *Re*covery does not mean unchanged. In fact, the victim might be extensively changed, psychologically as well as physically/physiologically. *Re*covery does connote a *re*-visioning, an attempt to get new meanings to line up with old ones [or global meanings, per Park and Kennedy (2016)] or to create new and modified ones. The *re*-building of meaning is a core issue of *re*storation and *re*covery and opens up hope for the future. The victim goes forward with new meanings that, according to Altmaier (2016), "serve in a developmental transformative way, shaking apart and reforming our lives through our perceptions, our constructions, our responses to both positive and negative events" (p. xvi).

Trauma and PTSD are biopsychosocial, spiritual, and contextual experiences. The job of therapists as healers is to address their clients in all of these dimensions and to help them address and integrate what was avoided. In doing so and in highly idiosyncratic ways, the clients develop a personal narrative that is one of interruption but one that is whole and personal nonetheless. They recuperate from what was lost or changed by the trauma and they renew their hope and reclaim their future.

REFERENCES

Altmaier, E. (2016). Introduction. In E. Altmaier (Ed.), *Reconstructing meaning after trauma*. San Diego, CA: Elsevier.

American Psychiatric Association. (2000). *Diagnostic and statistical manual of mental disorders* (Revised 4th ed.). Washington, DC: Author.

American Psychiatric Association. (2013). *Diagnostic and statistical manual of mental disorders 5*. Washington, DC: Author.

Freyd, J. (1998). *Betrayal-trauma: The logic of forgetting childhood abuse*. Boston: Harvard University Press.

Jay, J. (November/December 1991). Terrible knowledge. *Family Therapy Networker*, 19–29.

Kira, I. A. (2010). Etiology and treatment of post-cumulative traumatic stress disorders in different cultures. *Traumatology, 4*, 128–141.

Lifson, R. J. (1979). *The broken connection: On death and the continuity of life*. New York: Simon & Schuster.

Park, C. L., & Kennedy, M. C. (2016). Meaning violation and restoration following trauma: conceptual overview and clinical implications. In E. Altmeier (Ed.), *Reconstructing meaning after trauma*. San Diego, CA: Elsevier.

Putnam, F. W. (1997). *Dissociation in children and adolescents: A developmental perspective*. New York: Guilford Press.

Van der Hart, O., Nijenhuis, E. R. S., & Steele, K. (2006). *The haunted self: Structural dissociation and the treatment of chronic traumatization*. New York: W. W. Norton.

Wilson, J. P. (1989). *Trauma, transformation, and healing*. New York: Brunner/Mazel.

Yehuda, R. (Ed.). (1999). *Risk factors for posttraumatic stress disorders*. Washington, DC: American Psychiatric Press.

INDEX

'Note: Page numbers followed by "f" indicate figures and "t" indicate tables.'

Printed and bound by CPI Group (UK) Ltd, Croydon, CR0 4YY

08/06/2025

01896872-0009